AGING LIKE A SUPERSTAR

SECRETS TO TIMELESS BEAUTY AND VIBRANT HEALTH

ELLIOTT MIDDLETON PHD

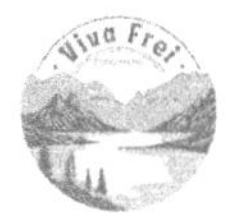

INTRODUCTION

Some years ago, I found myself standing in front of the bathroom mirror, scrutinizing the fine lines that had begun to etch themselves around my eyes. I wasn't exactly sure when they had first appeared, but they had been there for a while, undeniable and uninvited. My initial reaction was a mix of surprise and frustration, a far cry from the calm acceptance I had always imagined I would feel when this moment arrived. As I stood there, grappling with the reality of aging, a memory flashed through my mind—a moment of realization that would shape my journey from that point forward.

It was a quiet afternoon in Tennessee, where I had moved twenty years ago to embrace a slower, more intentional pace of life. I was walking along a wooded trail near my home, the golden light of the setting sun filtering through the trees, casting a warm glow on everything around me. I stopped to rest on a bench and found myself in the company of an older woman who told me she lived nearby. Her silver-blonde hair flowed down to her shoulders, and her eyes sparkled with a wisdom and serenity that immediately drew me in.

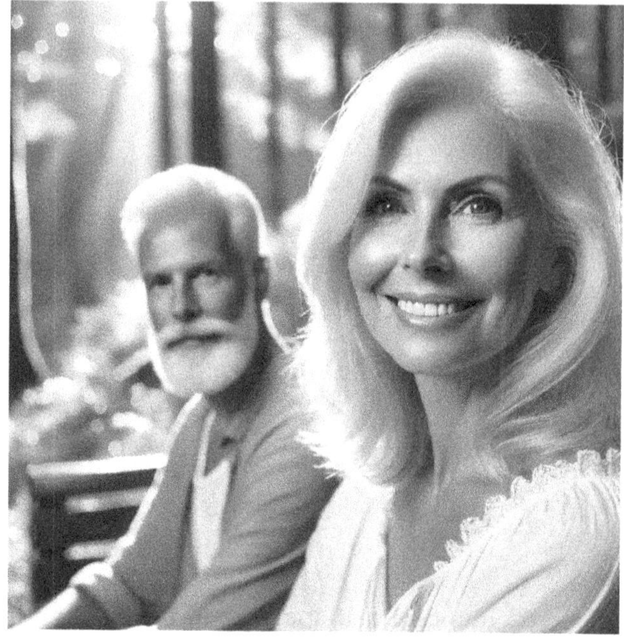

We talked for a while, and as we did, she shared her thoughts on aging with me. "It's not about holding on to the past," she said gently. "It's about embracing each new day, each new stage, with grace and gratitude. The lines on my face are just a map of the life I've lived—and I wouldn't trade them for anything."

That conversation stayed with me, echoing in my mind as I continued my walk and long after I returned home. It was a moment of clarity, a realization that aging isn't something to resist or fear but rather a journey to be embraced. And it was that realization that inspired me to write this book.

My name is Elliott Middleton, PhD. I'm a former university professor and decision scientist who spent years working in leading financial institutions. My career was demanding, often leaving little time for personal reflection or self-care. But as I transitioned into this new phase of life, I realized the importance of taking a holistic approach to aging—one that honors the mind, body, and spirit.

I've always firmly believed in the power of science, but I also recognize the value of natural remedies and the wisdom that comes with experience. My journey of aging gracefully here in Tennessee has been shaped by this blend of modern science and time-honored traditions, and it's a journey I'm eager to share with you.

The purpose of this book is simple: to provide a comprehensive, practical guide for women over 50 on how to age gracefully. But more than that, it's about empowering you to live with vitality, confidence, and joy in every aspect of your life. Whether you're looking for ways to maintain your physical health, nurture your mental well-being, or navigate life's transitions with poise, this book offers a holistic approach to help you thrive.

This book is designed for women like you—women over 50 who are ready to embrace this stage of life with open arms. You may be affluent or middle-class, accustomed to seeking quality information and products that enhance your life. You'll likely buy a paperback from Amazon, looking for something that speaks directly to your needs and aspirations. This book is tailored specifically for you, offering insights and advice that resonate with your experiences and challenges.

This book contains a wealth of information organized into carefully structured chapters with meticulous references. We'll begin by exploring the power of positivity and mindset, setting the foundation for aging with grace. From there, we'll delve into nutrition and holistic health, offering guidance on nourishing your body from the inside out. We'll discuss the importance of staying physically active with fitness routines designed for women over 50. Mental well-being will also be a key focus as we explore strategies for maintaining cognitive health and emotional balance.

Life transitions, whether they involve career changes, family dynamics, or personal growth, will be addressed with compassion and practical advice. We'll also touch on spiritual wellness, helping you connect with a unique sense of purpose and fulfillment. Finally, we'll offer practical lifestyle tips that make everyday living more joyful and satisfying.

By the end of this book, you'll have gained actionable advice, relatable stories, and empowering strategies to enhance your quality of life. I hope you'll learn to age gracefully and do so with excitement and anticipation for what lies ahead.

So, I invite you to dive in, engage fully with the content, and apply the tips and strategies that resonate with you. Aging is not the end of the journey—it's simply a new chapter filled with opportunities for growth, discovery, and joy. Let's embrace this stage of life together with grace, confidence, and an open heart.

Welcome to *Aging Like a Superstar!* Let the journey begin.

1

EMBRACING A GRACEFUL MINDSET

The Power of Positivity: Embracing Aging with Grace

Aging is inevitable, but how we perceive and approach it can make all the difference. Maintaining a positive attitude toward aging is not just a matter of feeling good—it's crucial for our emotional, mental, and even physical health. A positive mindset can transform how we experience aging, turning what many see as a decline into a journey of growth and self-discovery (Levy et al., 2002).

Reduced Stress Levels

Positivity acts as a powerful buffer against stress. When we approach life with a positive outlook, we're better equipped to handle challenges related to aging. Stress is often linked to adverse health outcomes, from heart disease to weakened immune function. By cultivating a positive attitude, we can reduce stress and its harmful effects on our bodies (Fredrickson, 2001).

Improved Physical Health

A positive mindset has been shown to improve physical health in numerous ways. People with a positive outlook are likelier to engage in healthy behaviors like regular exercise and balanced eating. They also tend to recover more quickly from illness and injury. The mind-body connection is strong; when we think positively, our bodies respond positively (Steptoe et al., 2009).

Better Relationships

Maintaining solid and healthy relationships becomes even more critical as we age. A positive attitude can help us navigate the changes in our social circles, whether adapting to new roles within our families or making new friends. Positivity fosters empathy, understanding, and communication—all vital to lasting relationships (Baumeister & Leary, 1995).

Increased Life Satisfaction

Aging with a positive attitude leads to greater life satisfaction. When we embrace the changes that come with age and focus on the joys rather than the losses, we open ourselves up to new experiences and opportunities. Life satisfaction isn't about having everything go perfectly; it's about finding contentment and joy in our lives (Wrosch et al., 2005).

Daily Affirmations

One practical way to foster a positive mindset is through daily affirmations. These are simple, powerful statements you repeat to reinforce positive beliefs and attitudes. Starting your day with affirmations can set the tone for the hours ahead, helping you focus on the positive aspects of your life (Emmons & McCullough, 2003).

Here are a few daily affirmations you can use to begin each day with positivity:

- **"I am grateful for my body and the experiences it has given me."**

Gratitude is a powerful tool for positivity. By acknowledging the strength and resilience of your body, you can appreciate the journey it has taken you on rather than focusing on any perceived flaws (Fredrickson, 2001).

- **"I embrace the wisdom that comes with age."**

With age comes wisdom—a deeper understanding of life, others, and ourselves. Embrace the knowledge and experience you've gained and recognize it as a valuable asset (Levy et al., 2002).

- **"Every day is an opportunity for growth and joy."**

Each day brings new possibilities. By viewing each day as an opportunity, you open yourself to experiences that can bring happiness and personal growth (Emmons & McCullough, 2003).

Overcoming Negative Thoughts

Even with the best intentions, negative thoughts can creep in. It's natural to experience self-doubt or concern about aging, but it's essential to recognize and combat these thoughts before they take root.

Cognitive-Behavioral Techniques

Cognitive-behavioral therapy (CBT) offers practical tools for identifying and changing negative thought patterns. When a negative thought arises—such as "I'm too old to try new things"—CBT encourages you to challenge that thought. Ask yourself: Is this thought based on facts? What evidence do I have that contradicts this belief? Over time, you can change your mindset by reframing negative thoughts into positive or neutral ones (Hofmann et al., 2012).

Journaling to Track Negative Thoughts

Writing down your thoughts can be a powerful way to understand and manage them. Keep a journal where you note any negative thoughts that arise, along with the situations that trigger them. Over time, you may notice patterns that can help you understand why these thoughts occur and how to address them (Pennebaker, 1997).

Replacing Negative Thoughts with Positive Affirmations

When a negative thought pops up, immediately counter it with a positive affirmation. For example, if you think, "I'm not as capable as I used to be," replace it with, "I am capable and have the wisdom to handle anything that comes my way." Over time, this practice can shift your thinking from negative to positive (Hofmann et al., 2012).

Inspirational Quotes

Sometimes, the words of others can provide the motivation and inspiration we need to keep a positive outlook on aging. Here are a few quotes from women who have embraced aging with grace and wisdom:

- **Maya Angelou:** "We delight in the beauty of the butterfly, but rarely admit the changes it has gone through to achieve that beauty."

This quote reminds us that aging is a process of transformation, and each stage of life brings its beauty and value (Angelou, 1994).

- **Helen Mirren:** "Aging is a wonderful thing. The older you get, the more you know, the more you realize that you don't know."

Helen Mirren's words capture the wisdom that comes with age—an understanding that life is about continuous learning and growth (Mirren, 2016).

- **Audrey Hepburn:** "The beauty of a woman with passing years only grows."

Hepburn's quote emphasizes that true beauty is timeless and grows stronger with age (Hepburn, 1991).

By embracing positivity, practicing daily affirmations, overcoming negative thoughts, and finding inspiration in the words of others, you can navigate the aging process with grace, joy, and confidence. Aging gracefully isn't about denying the years but embracing them with an open heart and a positive spirit.

Reframing Aging: Turning Challenges into Opportunities

Aging is often viewed as a series of challenges—physical changes, shifting social dynamics, and the inevitable passage of time. But what if, instead of seeing these challenges as obstacles, we viewed them as opportunities? Opportunities to grow, learn, and embrace life's fullness with a renewed sense of purpose and joy. Reframing how we think about aging can be transformative, allowing us to see the beauty in every stage of life (Carstensen et al., 2011).

Mindset Shifts

The first step in turning the challenges of aging into opportunities is to shift your mindset. Our thoughts and beliefs shape our experiences, and by consciously choosing to see aging through a positive lens, we can transform how we feel about it (Seligman, 2002).

Viewing Wrinkles as Signs of Wisdom and Experience

Wrinkles are often seen as the first visible signs of aging; for many, they can be a source of concern. But instead of viewing wrinkles as imperfections, try to see them as symbols of a life well-lived. Each line and crease tells a story—of laughter shared, challenges overcome, and lessons learned. They are marks of wisdom and experience and honor badges reflecting the depth and richness of your journey (Furman, 1997).

Seeing Retirement as a Time for New Adventures

Retirement is another aspect of aging that can be met with mixed emotions. For some, it signifies the end of a productive career, leaving a void that can be difficult to fill. However, retirement also offers a unique opportunity to explore new interests and passions. It's a time to rediscover what brings you joy, travel, learn new skills, and engage in activities you may not have had time for. Rather than seeing retirement as the end of an era, embrace it as the beginning of a new adventure (Atchley, 1989).

Storytelling

One of the most powerful ways to inspire change is through storytelling. Real-life stories of women who have successfully reframed their aging process can serve as motivating examples of what is possible when we shift our perspective.

A Woman Who Started a New Career at 60

Meet Susan, a woman who, at 60, decided it was time for a change. After decades of working in the corporate world, she retired and felt restless. Rather than settle into a leisure routine, Susan pursued a passion she had long put on hold—writing. She enrolled in a creative writing course, and with determination and creativity, she authored her first novel within two years. That novel became a bestseller, launching a new career for Susan as an author. Her story is a testament to the idea that it's never too late to chase your dreams or start something new (Levine, 2004).

Someone Who Took Up a New Hobby and Excelled

Then there's Martha, who, at 65, decided to take up painting—a hobby she had always been curious about but never had the time to explore. She started with a beginner's class at her local community center, and what began as a simple pastime quickly blossomed into a passion. Over the years, Martha's skills improved, and her work began to attract attention. She eventually held her first art exhibition at 70, where several paintings were sold. Martha's journey illustrates how embracing new interests can lead to unexpected fulfillment and recognition (Csikszentmihalyi, 1997).

Practical Exercises

Here are some practical exercises you can start today to help you reframe your thoughts about aging and turn challenges into opportunities.

Gratitude Journaling

Gratitude is a powerful tool for reframing your mindset. Start a gratitude journal where you write down three things you're grateful for daily, focusing on aspects of aging that you appreciate. This could be the wisdom you've gained over the years, the time you now have to pursue hobbies or the joy of watching your family grow. By consistently focusing on the positives, you'll begin to reframe how you see aging naturally (Emmons & McCullough, 2003).

Vision Boards

Creating a vision board is another effective way to shift your mindset and focus on the opportunities that come with aging. Gather images, quotes, and symbols representing the life you want to create in this stage. Whether it's pictures of places you want to travel, hobbies you want to pursue, or even words that inspire you, placing these visual reminders in a space where you'll see them daily can help keep your mind focused on the possibilities rather than the limitations (Locke & Latham, 2002).

Benefits of Reframing

The benefits of adopting a positive outlook on aging are profound, impacting both your emotional and psychological well-being.

Reduced Anxiety and Stress

When you shift your perspective and see aging as a journey full of opportunities, the anxiety and stress that often accompany aging can diminish. Instead of worrying about what's to come, you'll look forward to it, naturally reducing stress levels. A positive outlook can also make it easier to cope with the inevitable changes that aging brings, as you'll be more inclined to see them as part of the natural progression of life (Fredrickson, 2001).

Increased Happiness and Fulfillment

The most significant benefit of reframing aging is the increase in overall happiness and fulfillment. By focusing on the opportunities rather than the challenges, you can cultivate a more profound sense of satisfaction with your life. You'll find joy in the present moment and excitement for the future, contributing to a more fulfilled, contented life (Wrosch et al., 2005).

Reframing Aging is not about denying the challenges—it's about choosing to focus on the opportunities that come with them. By shifting your mindset, embracing new possibilities, and practicing gratitude, you can transform your aging experience into one of growth, joy, and fulfillment. Aging gracefully is not just about maintaining physical appearance or health; it's about nurturing a positive, empowered mindset that allows you to live your best life at any age.

Cultivating Gratitude: Daily Practices for a Positive Outlook

Gratitude is more than just a fleeting emotion; it's a powerful tool that can transform your outlook on life, especially as you age. Cultivating a daily gratitude practice can enhance mental and emotional health, creating a positive ripple effect. By consciously focusing on what you are thankful for, you can foster a mindset that appreciates the present and embraces the future with optimism (Emmons & McCullough, 2003).

The Science of Gratitude

The idea that gratitude can improve your well-being isn't just a feel-good concept; it's backed by solid scientific research. Studies have shown that people who regularly practice gratitude experience various psychological and emotional benefits.

Studies Showing Increased Happiness

Research has consistently found a strong correlation between gratitude and happiness. In one study conducted by Dr. Robert

Emmons, a leading expert on gratitude, participants who kept a weekly gratitude journal reported feeling more optimistic and satisfied with their lives than those who didn't. They also exercised more and had fewer visits to the doctor, indicating that gratitude can have tangible effects on physical health (Emmons & McCullough, 2003).

Lower Levels of Depression

Research shows that gratitude practice also reduces symptoms of depression. In a study published in the *Journal of Psychosomatic Research*, individuals who practiced gratitude experienced lower levels of depression and higher levels of overall well-being. Focusing on positive aspects of life, even small ones, can counteract negative thought patterns and promote a more balanced, positive mindset (Wood et al., 2010).

Understanding the science behind gratitude makes it clear that this practice is not just a fleeting trend but a foundational aspect of mental and emotional health. Incorporating gratitude into daily life can significantly enhance your well-being (Emmons & McCullough, 2003).

Gratitude Journaling

One of the most effective ways to cultivate gratitude is through journaling. A gratitude journal is a simple yet powerful tool that helps you regularly focus on the positive aspects of your life. Here's how you can structure your gratitude journaling practice:

Daily Prompts

To help you get started, use specific prompts that encourage you to think deeply about what you're grateful for. Here are a few examples:

- What are three things that happened today that I'm grateful for?
- Who is someone in my life that I'm thankful for, and why?
- What challenge did I face today, and what did I learn from it?

These prompts will help you reflect on your day and identify moments of gratitude, even amid challenges (Emmons & McCullough, 2003).

Reflective Questions

Besides daily prompts, consider adding reflective questions to your journaling practice. These questions encourage deeper introspection and can help you uncover areas of your life that you might otherwise overlook:

- How has gratitude influenced my mood or perspective today?
- What small things brought me joy today, and how can I incorporate more of them into my life?
- In what ways can I express my gratitude to others?

By answering these questions, you can better understand how gratitude impacts your life and how you can continue cultivating it (Emmons & McCullough, 2003).

Daily Gratitude Practices

Beyond journaling, you can incorporate several simple daily practices into your routine to cultivate a grateful mindset.

Morning Gratitude Meditation

Starting your day with a gratitude meditation can set a positive tone for the hours ahead. Find a quiet space, close your eyes, and take a few deep breaths. As you breathe, focus on what you're grateful for —whether it's the comfort of your bed, the warmth of the sun, or the presence of loved ones. This practice doesn't need to be long; even five minutes of focused gratitude in the morning can significantly affect your outlook for the day (Fredrickson, 2001).

Thank-You Notes

Another simple but impactful practice is writing thank-you notes. Take a few moments each week to write a note to someone who has positively impacted your life. It doesn't have to be elaborate—a short, heartfelt message is enough to express your gratitude. Whether it's a friend, family member, or even a colleague, these notes strengthen your relationships and reinforce your appreciation (Emmons & McCullough, 2003).

Gratitude in Relationships

Expressing gratitude benefits you and strengthens your relationships with others. When you show appreciation for the people in your life, you create a positive environment that fosters connection and understanding (Algoe et al., 2010).

Verbal Affirmations to Loved Ones

One of the simplest ways to express gratitude in relationships is through verbal affirmations. Make it a habit to tell your loved ones how much they mean to you. Whether you thank your partner for their support, acknowledge a friend for their kindness, or express appreciation to a family member for their love, these affirmations can deepen your bonds and create a more positive, supportive dynamic (Algoe et al., 2010).

Acts of Kindness

Gratitude can also be expressed through actions. Consider performing small acts of kindness for those around you—making a loved one's favorite meal, helping a neighbor with a task, or simply offering a listening ear. These actions demonstrate your appreciation and can significantly enhance your relationships, creating a cycle of positivity and gratitude (Emmons & McCullough, 2003).

Benefits of Reframing

As you cultivate gratitude daily, you'll notice this practice's profound emotional and psychological benefits.

Reduced Anxiety and Stress

Gratitude helps shift your focus away from what's lacking or what's wrong, reducing feelings of anxiety and stress. When you concentrate on the positive aspects of your life, you naturally create a more peaceful and content state of mind, which can lower stress and anxiety levels (Fredrickson, 2001).

Increased Happiness and Fulfillment

Consistent gratitude leads to increased happiness and a greater sense of fulfillment. By regularly acknowledging the good in your life, you create a habit of positivity that permeates all aspects of your existence. This enhances your day-to-day experiences and contributes to a more profound sense of life satisfaction (Emmons & McCullough, 2003).

Cultivating gratitude is a powerful way to enhance your quality of life, especially as you age. By incorporating these daily practices—journaling, meditation, or expressing gratitude in your relationships—you can foster a positive outlook that improves your mental and emotional health and enriches your connections with others. Gratitude is a simple yet transformative practice that can help you embrace aging with grace, joy, and a deep sense of fulfillment.

Building Resilience: Bouncing Back from Life's Setbacks

Life is full of unexpected challenges, which can sometimes feel more daunting as we age. Whether it's a health issue, a significant life change, or an emotional setback, the ability to bounce back—resilience—becomes increasingly important. Resilience is not about avoiding difficulties but how we respond to them. It's about cultivating the inner strength to navigate life's ups and downs with grace and perseverance (Bonanno, 2004).

Defining Resilience

Resilience is the ability to "bounce back" from adversity, but it's much more than that. It's about emotional elasticity—the capacity to stretch and adapt in the face of challenges and to return to a state of balance after a setback. Resilience involves adaptability, allowing us to adjust our mindset, behaviors, and actions to better cope with changes and difficulties (Southwick et al., 2014).

Emotional Elasticity

Emotional elasticity refers to the ability to manage and recover from emotional distress. It's the capacity to experience various emotions—anger, sadness, frustration—without being overwhelmed. This flexibility allows us to process our feelings, learn from our experiences, and emerge more robust and grounded (Tugade & Fredrickson, 2004).

Adaptability

Adaptability is adjusting to new circumstances, whether unexpected changes in our personal lives, health, or broader societal shifts. As we age, adaptability becomes crucial, enabling us to navigate the inevitable transitions that come with growing older. It's about being open to change and finding ways to thrive in new and different situations (Southwick et al., 2014).

Strategies for Building Resilience

Building resilience is a lifelong process that involves cultivating specific habits and mindsets. Here are some practical strategies to help you develop and strengthen your resilience:

Mindfulness and Meditation

Mindfulness is being fully present in the moment, without judgment. It helps you become more aware of your thoughts and emotions, allowing you to respond to challenges with greater clarity and calmness. Meditation is a powerful tool for cultivating mindfulness. Even a few minutes of daily meditation can help you develop the mental discipline to manage stress and build resilience. Techniques such as mindful breathing, body scans, or guided imagery can be especially effective in helping you stay centered during difficult times (Kabat-Zinn, 2003).

Physical Activity

Physical activity is essential for maintaining your physical health and building resilience. Regular exercise releases endorphins, natural mood enhancers, and helps reduce stress. It also improves your overall energy levels and mental clarity. Activities like yoga, walking, swimming, or any form of exercise that you enjoy can help you develop the strength and stamina to handle life's challenges more effectively (Salmon, 2001).

Seeking Social Support

Building and maintaining strong social connections is crucial to resilience. A supportive network of friends, family, or community members provides emotional support, practical assistance, and a sense of belonging. Don't hesitate to reach out when you need help, whether it's just someone to talk to or more tangible forms of support. Engaging in social activities, volunteering, or joining groups that align with your interests can also help you build a resilient support network (Cohen & Wills, 1985).

Resilience in Action

It's helpful to see resilience in action to truly understand it. Here are stories of women who have demonstrated remarkable resilience in the face of adversity, showing that they can survive challenges and thrive because of them.

Overcoming Health Challenges

Consider the story of Jane, who was diagnosed with a severe illness in her late 50s. Initially, the news was devastating, and Jane struggled with fear and uncertainty about her future. However, she decided to approach her illness with a resilient mindset. She educated herself about her condition, sought out the best possible care, and committed to a healthy lifestyle that included diet changes, regular exercise, and stress management techniques like yoga and meditation. Jane also leaned on her friends and family for support, allowing herself to be vulnerable and accepting help when needed. Today, Jane is not only managing her illness but has also become an advocate for others facing similar challenges, proving that resilience can turn even the most difficult situations into opportunities for growth and contribution (Bonanno, 2004).

Navigating Significant Life Changes

Another example is Linda, who faced the unexpected loss of her spouse after 40 years of marriage. The grief was overwhelming, and Linda found herself at a crossroads, unsure of how to move forward. Instead of being consumed by sadness, Linda chose to rebuild her life in a way that honored her past while embracing the future. She began by focusing on self-care, taking up new hobbies like painting and gardening, and reconnecting with old friends. Linda also started volunteering at a local community center and found a new sense of purpose and fulfillment. Through these actions, she navigated her profound loss with resilience, eventually finding joy and meaning in her new life (Neimeyer, 2000).

Daily Resilience Practices

You cultivate resilience through daily habits and practices that strengthen your emotional and mental fortitude. Here are some simple, effective practices you can incorporate into your daily routine to build and maintain resilience:

Mindful Breathing Exercises

Mindful breathing is a simple yet powerful way to calm your mind and build resilience. Take a few moments each day to focus on your breath. Inhale deeply through your nose, allowing your abdomen to expand, then exhale slowly through your mouth. As you breathe, pay attention to the sensation of the air entering and leaving your body. This practice can help you manage stress, clear your mind, and center yourself, making it easier to respond to life's challenges with resilience (Kabat-Zinn, 2003).

Reflective Journaling

Journaling is another effective way to build resilience. Set aside time daily to reflect on your experiences, thoughts, and emotions. Write about your challenges and how you've responded to them. This practice allows you to process your feelings, gain insights into your behavior, and track your progress over time. Regularly reflecting on your resilience reinforces your ability to bounce back from setbacks and approach future challenges more confidently (Pennebaker, 1997).

Building resilience is an ongoing process that requires intentional effort, but the rewards are well worth it. By developing emotional elasticity and adaptability and engaging in daily resilience practices, you can navigate life's inevitable challenges with grace and strength. Resilience helps you bounce back from adversity and empowers you to live a fuller, more meaningful life at any age (Southwick et al., 2014).

Finding Your Purpose: Staying Motivated in Your Later Years

As we move into the later stages of life, finding and maintaining a sense of purpose becomes increasingly essential. Purpose gives our lives direction and meaning, fueling our motivation and contributing significantly to our mental and emotional well-being. It's not uncommon to feel a sense of loss or uncertainty about purpose as you age, especially after significant life changes like retirement or the departure of grown children. However, these years can also be a time of incredible growth and fulfillment as you discover new passions and set goals that align with your evolving sense of self (Hill & Turiano, 2014).

Importance of Purpose

A clear sense of purpose is essential for maintaining a positive outlook on life, especially as you age. Purpose acts as a guiding star, providing direction and motivation that helps you navigate both daily routines and life's challenges (McKnight & Kashdan, 2009).

Increased Motivation

When you have a strong sense of purpose, waking up each day with enthusiasm and determination becomes easier. Purpose-driven individuals are more likely to engage in activities that are meaningful to them, which in turn boosts their motivation and energy levels. Whether pursuing a new hobby, volunteering, or working on personal goals, a clear sense of purpose can inspire you to take action and stay committed (Steger et al., 2008).

Higher Levels of Happiness

Purpose is closely linked to happiness and life satisfaction. Studies have shown that people with a strong sense of purpose experience higher happiness and fulfillment. Purpose provides a sense of accomplishment and contribution, making life more meaningful. Living purposefully makes you more likely to experience joy in significant achievements and small daily tasks, leading to a richer and more satisfying life (Hill & Turiano, 2014).

Discovering Your Passion

Finding your purpose begins with identifying your passions—those activities, causes, or pursuits that ignite your enthusiasm and bring you joy. If you're not sure where your passions lie, here are some exercises that can help you discover them:

Passion Questionnaires

A passion questionnaire helps uncover what excites and motivates you. Try answering the following questions to get a clearer sense of your passions:

- What activities or topics do I find myself naturally drawn to?
- What tasks make me lose track of time because I'm so engaged?
- What causes or issues do I feel strongly about?
- When was the last time I felt truly fulfilled, and what was I doing?

Reflecting on these questions can help you identify recurring themes or interests pointing to your passions. Once you've identified these, you can explore more ways to incorporate them into your life (Hill & Turiano, 2014).

Reflection on Past Experiences

Another effective way to discover your passions is to reflect on past experiences that brought you joy or satisfaction. Think about moments when you felt alive, engaged, and fulfilled. What were you doing? Who were you with? What was the context? These memories can provide valuable clues about what activities or environments resonate most with you. Use these insights to guide your exploration of new or renewed passions in your later years (McKnight & Kashdan, 2009).

Setting Goals

Once you've identified your passions, the next step is to set goals that align with them. Goal setting is essential to living with purpose, as it gives you specific objectives to work toward and helps you measure your progress.

SMART Goals Framework

The SMART goals framework is a popular and effective method for setting Specific, Measurable, Achievable, Relevant, and Time-bound goals. Here's how you can apply the SMART framework to your goals:

• **Specific:** Clearly define what you want to achieve. For example, instead of saying, "I want to get fit," specify, "I want to walk 30 minutes daily."

• **Measurable:** Establish criteria for measuring your progress. If you want to write a book, set milestones like "complete one chapter per month."

• **Achievable:** Set goals that are challenging but realistic. Consider your current abilities and resources, and ensure your goals are within reach.

• **Relevant:** Align your goals with your passions and purpose. Choose goals that are meaningful to you and that contribute to your overall sense of fulfillment.

• **Time-bound:** Set a deadline for achieving your goals. Deadlines help create a sense of urgency and motivate you to stay on track (Locke & Latham, 2002).

By following the SMART framework, you can create realistic and fulfilling goals to help you stay motivated and purpose-driven.

Long-term vs. Short-term Goals

It's crucial to balance long-term goals with short-term ones. Long-term goals, like learning a new language or starting a nonprofit, give you something significant to work toward over time. Short-term goals, like reading a book each month or completing a craft project, provide more immediate satisfaction and help you build momentum. Together, these goals ensure you're continually progressing and staying engaged (Steger et al., 2008).

Living with Purpose

Living with purpose means actively pursuing the goals and passions that bring meaning to your life. Here are some real-life examples of women who have found new purposes in their later years, demonstrating that it's never too late to live purpose-driven lives.

Volunteering Stories

Consider Margaret, who, after retiring from a long career in education, found herself missing the daily interactions with students and colleagues. Instead of seeing retirement as the end of her teaching journey, Margaret began volunteering at a local literacy program, helping adults learn to read. This new role allowed her to continue making a difference and introduced her to a vibrant community of like-minded individuals. Volunteering gave Margaret a renewed sense of purpose, and she now describes this chapter of her life as one of the most rewarding (Morrow-Howell et al., 2003).

New Career or Hobby Pursuits

Then there's Nancy, who discovered her passion for gardening later in life. What started as a simple backyard project blossomed into a full-fledged pursuit. Nancy took horticulture classes and eventually started a small business selling organic herbs and flowers at local markets. This new venture brought her joy, purpose, and even a new circle of friends who shared her love for gardening. Nancy's story is a powerful reminder that pursuing a new career or hobby that aligns with your passions is never too late (Csikszentmihalyi, 1997).

Finding and living purposefully in your later years can bring immense satisfaction, motivation, and joy. By discovering your passions, setting meaningful goals, and actively pursuing them, you can create a rich life with purpose and fulfillment. These years are not just about reflecting on the past—they are about embracing the present and future with intention, excitement, and a deep sense of purpose (McKnight & Kashdan, 2009).

The Joy of Lifelong Learning: Keeping Your Mind Sharp

One of the most rewarding and fulfilling pursuits we can embrace as we journey through life is the joy of lifelong learning. This isn't just about acquiring new information—it's about keeping our minds sharp, our spirits engaged, and our lives enriched with new experiences and insights. Learning doesn't have an expiration date, and as we grow older, it becomes even more important to stay curious, open, and excited about the world around us (Simonton, 2001).

Benefits of Lifelong Learning

Continuing to learn new things as we age is not just beneficial—it's essential. Learning keeps our brains active and healthy, offering cognitive and emotional benefits that can significantly enhance our quality of life (Hertzog et al., 2008).

Improved Memory

Learning new skills or absorbing new information challenges the brain, helping to maintain and even improve memory function. We work out our brains when we engage in activities requiring us to recall information, solve problems, or think creatively. Physical exercise strengthens our bodies, and mental exercise strengthens our minds, helping preserve memory and cognitive function as we age (Hertzog et al., 2008).

Enhanced Problem-Solving Skills

Learning isn't just about storing facts but thinking critically and solving problems. When you take on the challenge of learning something new, you acquire knowledge and enhance your ability to think analytically and creatively. You become more adept at handling life's complexities and challenges, giving you the tools to navigate new situations confidently and efficiently (Simonton, 2001).

Learning Opportunities

In today's world, there are more opportunities than ever to continue learning, regardless of age. Whether you prefer the convenience of online courses or the camaraderie of in-person classes, there's something out there for everyone. Here are a few options to consider:

Online Courses

The internet has opened up a world of learning opportunities you can access from the comfort of your home. Websites like Coursera, edX, and Udemy offer a vast array of courses on everything from history and literature to technology and personal development. Many of these courses are free or available at a low cost, and they allow you to learn at your own pace, making it easier to fit learning into your life (Means et al., 2010).

Community Classes

If you prefer a more social learning experience, consider enrolling. Local community centers, libraries, and adult education programs often offer courses in various subjects, from cooking and photography to language learning and computer skills. These classes provide a structured learning environment and an excellent opportunity to meet new people and build connections with others who share your interests (Simonton, 2001).

Book Clubs

For those who love to read, joining a book club can be a fantastic way to engage with new ideas and perspectives. Book clubs provide a platform to explore literature, discuss themes, and share insights with others. Whether you join a local club or participate in an online community, book clubs can deepen your understanding of the world and introduce you to genres and authors you might not have discovered (DeGarmo, 2010).

Engaging in New Hobbies

One of the most enjoyable ways to keep your mind sharp and your life rich with experiences is to take up new hobbies and interests. Hobbies provide mental stimulation, a sense of accomplishment, and joy as you develop new skills.

Learning a Musical Instrument

Playing a musical instrument is a beautiful way to engage your mind and emotions. Whether you've always wanted to play the piano, strum a guitar, or take up the violin, it's never too late to start. Learning an instrument challenges your brain, improving coordination, memory, and emotional expression. Making music is a profoundly satisfying and creative outlet (Bugos et al., 2007).

Gardening

Gardening is more than just a pastime—it's a way to connect with nature, nurture living things, and enjoy your labor's fruits (and flowers). Gardening can be incredibly therapeutic, offering physical activity, mental relaxation, and the joy of watching something grow. It's also a great way to learn about plants, ecosystems, and sustainable practices (Gross & Lane, 2007).

Painting

Painting can be a wonderfully fulfilling hobby whether you're an experienced artist or a beginner. It allows you to express yourself creatively, experiment with colors and techniques, and discover new things. Painting is also a fantastic way to relieve stress, focus your mind, and create something beautiful to enjoy and share with others (Simonton, 2001).

Sharing Knowledge

One of the greatest joys of learning is sharing what you've learned. Teaching, mentoring, or simply sharing your knowledge with friends and family can gratify you and those you're helping.

Teaching or Mentoring

If you have expertise or experience in a particular field, consider teaching or mentoring others through formal avenues like adult education classes or informal settings like community groups or one-on-one mentoring. Sharing your knowledge helps others, reinforces your understanding, and engages your mind (Booth et al., 2004).

Writing and Blogging

Writing is a powerful way to share your insights, experiences, and knowledge with a broader audience. Whether you're writing a memoir, a how-to guide, or a blog, putting your thoughts into words can be a fulfilling way to communicate your passions and connect with others. Blogging, in particular, offers the opportunity to reach a global audience and engage in meaningful conversations with readers from all walks of life (DeGarmo, 2010).

Lifelong learning is a critical component of aging gracefully. It keeps your mind sharp, your spirit engaged, and your life rich with meaning and purpose. By embracing the opportunities to learn through formal education, new hobbies, or sharing your knowledge with others, you can continue to grow and thrive at every stage of life. So, go ahead—explore, create, and share. The world is full of possibilities, and there's always something new to discover (Simonton, 2001).

2

NOURISHING YOUR BODY NATURALLY

Superfoods for Superwomen: Boosting Energy with Nutrition

As we age, our bodies undergo various changes that affect our energy levels, metabolism, and overall health. While these changes are natural, the good news is that our foods can significantly affect how we feel each day. Enter superfoods—nutrient-packed powerhouses that can help you boost energy, support overall health, and keep you feeling vibrant and strong. In this chapter, we'll explore the benefits of these superfoods and how you can easily incorporate them into your daily meals to enhance your well-being.

Introduction to Superfoods

The term "superfood" is often used to describe foods that are exceptionally rich in nutrients and offer a variety of health benefits in just one serving. While there is no strict scientific definition for superfoods, they include foods with high concentrations of vitamins, minerals, antioxidants, and other essential nutrients that support optimal health.

Antioxidant Properties: One critical feature of many superfoods is their antioxidant content. Antioxidants help protect your body from oxidative stress, which can lead to cellular damage and accelerate the aging process. By neutralizing free radicals, antioxidants can reduce the risk of chronic diseases, improve skin health, and even enhance cognitive function. For aging women, incorporating antioxidant-rich foods into your diet is a powerful way to support overall health and longevity.

Nutrient Density: Superfoods are also celebrated for their nutrient density, meaning they pack many essential vitamins, minerals, and other nutrients into relatively few calories. They are particularly beneficial for women over 50, who may need to focus on nutrient-rich foods to meet their dietary needs without consuming excessive calories. By choosing foods that are high in nutrients but low in empty calories, you can maintain energy levels, support bone health, and reduce the risk of age-related illnesses.

Anti-Inflammatory Effects: Chronic inflammation is a common issue that can lead to various health problems, including joint pain, cardiovascular disease, and digestive issues. Many superfoods have natural anti-inflammatory properties that can help reduce inflammation in the body, promoting better health and comfort as you age. Regularly consuming these foods can support your body's natural ability to heal and protect itself from inflammation.

Top Superfoods

Now that we've covered what makes superfoods so unique, let's take a closer look at some of the top superfoods that can boost your energy and overall health.

Blueberries: Rich in Antioxidants Blueberries are often at the top of the superfoods list, and for good reason. These small but mighty berries pack many antioxidants, particularly flavonoids, which protect the brain from oxidative stress and reduce the risk of cognitive decline. In addition to their brain-boosting benefits, blueberries are also high in vitamin C and fiber, making them an excellent choice for supporting immune health and digestion.

Kale: High in Vitamins A, C, and K Kale is a leafy green vegetable that has earned its reputation as a nutritional powerhouse. It's incredibly rich in vitamins A, C, and K—essential for eye health, immune function, and bone strength. Kale also contains antioxidants like quercetin and kaempferol, which have anti-inflammatory effects. Whether you enjoy it in salads, smoothies, or sautéed as a side dish, kale is a versatile superfood that can enhance your overall health.

Quinoa: Complete Protein Source Quinoa is a unique grain because it's one of the few plant-based foods considered a complete protein, meaning it contains all nine essential amino acids your body needs to build and repair tissues. Quinoa is an excellent choice for women looking to maintain muscle mass and strength as they age. Quinoa is also high in fiber, magnesium, and iron, supporting digestive health and energy production.

Chia Seeds: Omega-3 Fatty Acids Chia seeds may be tiny, but they pack large quantities of omega-3 fatty acids essential for heart health, brain function, and reducing inflammation. In addition to omega-3s, chia seeds are a good source of fiber and protein, helping to keep you full and satisfied. It is straightforward to incorporate these seeds into your diet—sprinkle them on your yogurt, blend them into smoothies, or make a simple chia seed pudding.

Incorporating Superfoods into Daily Meals

Incorporating superfoods into your daily meals doesn't have to be complicated. Here are some practical tips and delicious recipes to help you enjoy these nutrient-dense foods daily.

Smoothie Recipes with Spinach and Berries: One of the easiest ways to start your day with a burst of nutrition is by making a smoothie. Combine a handful of fresh spinach with a cup of mixed berries (including blueberries), a scoop of your favorite protein powder, and some almond milk or yogurt. Blend until smooth, and you have a quick, energizing breakfast loaded with antioxidants, vitamins, and protein.

Salad Recipes Featuring Kale and Quinoa: For a nutritious and satisfying lunch or dinner, try a salad that combines kale and quinoa. Start with a base of chopped kale, massage it with olive oil to soften the leaves, and then add cooked quinoa. Top your salad with cherry tomatoes, avocado slices, and a sprinkle of feta cheese. Drizzle with a lemon-tahini dressing, and you have a delicious meal rich in essential nutrients.

Chia Seed Pudding for Breakfast: Chia seed pudding is a simple and versatile breakfast option you can prepare the night before. Mix three tablespoons of chia seeds with one cup of almond milk, a teaspoon of honey or maple syrup, and a splash of vanilla extract. Stir well, cover, and refrigerate overnight. In the morning, you'll have a thick, creamy pudding topped with fresh berries, nuts, or a dollop of yogurt. It's a satisfying way to start your day with a boost of omega-3s and fiber.

Personal Stories and Testimonials

Hearing from women who have experienced the benefits of superfoods is helpful in truly understanding their power. Here are a few stories of how incorporating these nutrient-rich foods into their diets has changed their lives.

Increased Energy Levels: Joan, a 62-year-old retiree, started adding more superfoods to her diet after noticing her energy levels were dipping. "I began by making small changes—adding blueberries to my morning oatmeal and switching to quinoa instead of white rice," she says. "Within a few weeks, I noticed I had more energy throughout the day, and I wasn't as sluggish in the afternoons. It was a game-changer for me."

Improved Digestion and Skin Health: Linda, 58, found that incorporating chia seeds and kale into her diet improved her digestion and gave her skin a healthy glow. "I've struggled with digestive issues for years, but once I started eating more fiber-rich foods like chia seeds and leafy greens, I noticed a significant improvement," she shares. "And as a bonus, my skin looks better than it has in years—I'm convinced it's the antioxidants and nutrients from these superfoods."

These stories are a testament to the powerful impact that superfoods can have on your health and well-being. By making these foods a regular part of your diet, you can enjoy the benefits of increased energy, improved digestion, and overall vitality.

Hydration Habits: The Importance of Water and Hydrating Foods

Staying hydrated is a cornerstone of good health, and its importance becomes even more pronounced as we age. Water is essential for nearly every function in the body, from maintaining energy levels to supporting the health of your skin and joints. In this section, we'll explore why hydration is so crucial, how much water you should drink daily, and how to boost your hydration through fluids and foods.

Why Hydration Matters

Water is the body's most vital nutrient, and proper hydration is critical to keeping everything running smoothly. As we age, our bodies become less efficient at conserving water, making it even more important to be mindful of our hydration habits. Here's why staying hydrated matters:

Role in Digestion: Water plays a critical role in the digestive process. It helps break down food so that your body can absorb nutrients more effectively, and it aids in the smooth movement of food through your digestive tract. Proper hydration can prevent constipation, a common issue that can become more prevalent as we age. Consuming enough water can help keep your digestive system functioning optimally, reducing discomfort and improving overall well-being.

Impact on Skin Health: As we grow older, our skin naturally loses moisture, leading to dryness, wrinkles, and a less supple appearance. Staying well-hydrated can help combat these effects by keeping your skin hydrated from within. Water helps maintain skin elasticity and can reduce the appearance of fine lines. While hydration alone won't eliminate wrinkles, it's a simple and effective way to support your skin's health and maintain a youthful glow.

Importance for Joint Lubrication: Hydration is also crucial for joint health. Water makes up a significant portion of the synovial fluid that lubricates your joints, allowing them to move smoothly and without pain. As you age, joint pain and stiffness can become more common, but staying hydrated can help keep your joints well-lubricated and reduce discomfort. Keeping your joints healthy is essential for maintaining mobility and enjoying an active lifestyle.

Daily Water Intake Recommendations

So, how much water should you be drinking each day? The answer can vary depending on several factors, including your activity level, climate, and overall health.

General Recommendations: Drinking about 8 cups (64 ounces) of water daily is a standard guideline and a good baseline for most people. This helps ensure your body stays hydrated. You may need more or less, depending on your individual needs.

Adjustments for Activity Level and Climate: If you're physically active, your body will lose more water through sweat, so increasing your water intake is vital to compensate. Similarly, if you live in a hot or humid climate, you'll need to drink more water to stay hydrated. A good rule of thumb is to drink an additional cup of water for every 30 minutes of exercise or if you're spending extended time in the sun. Remember, your body constantly loses water, even when you're not exercising, so staying mindful of hydration is critical to maintaining good health.

Hydrating Foods

While drinking water is the most direct way to stay hydrated, you can also boost your hydration by eating foods with a high water content. These foods help you stay hydrated and provide additional health benefits thanks to their nutrient content.

Cucumbers: High Water Content and Vitamins: Cucumbers comprise about 95% water, making them one of the most hydrating foods you can eat. They're also low in calories and vitamins C and K, supporting skin health and bone strength. Slicing cucumbers into your salads or snacking on them throughout the day is an easy and refreshing way to increase your water intake.

Watermelon: Hydrating and Rich in Antioxidants: Watermelon is another hydrating food containing about 92% water. It's also rich in antioxidants like lycopene, which can help protect your cells from damage. Enjoying a slice of watermelon on a hot day is delicious and an excellent way to hydrate and get a dose of vitamins A and C.

Celery: Hydrating and Low in Calories: Celery is about 95% water and incredibly low in calories, making it an excellent snack for those looking to maintain a healthy weight while staying hydrated. Celery also contains fiber, which supports digestive health, and it's a good source of vitamin K, which is essential for blood clotting and bone health.

Creative Hydration Tips

Drinking enough water each day can sometimes feel like a chore, but it doesn't have to be. Here are some creative tips to make hydration more enjoyable and achievable:

Infused Water Recipes with Fruits and Herbs: If plain water feels boring, try infusing it with fruits and herbs for a refreshing twist. Add slices of citrus fruits like lemon or lime, berries, cucumber, or fresh herbs like mint or basil to a water pitcher. Let it sit for a few hours in the fridge to allow the flavors to meld, and you'll have a delicious, naturally flavored water that's a pleasure to drink.

Setting Hydration Reminders on Smartphones: In the hustle and bustle of daily life, it's easy to forget to drink water. Setting reminders on your smartphone can help you stay on track. Many apps are available that can gently nudge you throughout the day, reminding you to take a sip. You can also set alarms at specific times, like every hour, to ensure you're regularly hydrating.

Using a Hydration Tracking App: If you like to keep track of your habits, using a hydration tracking app can be a great way to monitor your water intake. These apps allow you to log how much water you drink each day and can provide insights into your hydration habits. Some apps even offer personalized recommendations based on your activity level and climate, making it easier to stay hydrated and healthy.

Staying hydrated is one of the simplest yet most effective ways to support your health as you age. By drinking enough water, eating hydrating foods, and incorporating creative strategies to make hydration a habit, you can keep your body functioning at its best. Remember, hydration isn't just about quenching your thirst—it's about nourishing your entire body, from your skin and joints to your digestion and beyond.

DIY Natural Skincare: Recipes for Glowing Skin

Caring for your skin is one of the most important aspects of aging gracefully. As more people become aware of the potential drawbacks of synthetic skincare products, natural skincare has gained popularity. Natural ingredients nourish the skin and offer a gentle, effective way to maintain a healthy, radiant complexion without exposing your body to harsh chemicals. In this section, we'll explore the benefits of natural skincare, introduce you to essential DIY ingredients, share some simple and practical recipes, and offer tips on establishing a skincare routine to keep your skin glowing.

Benefits of Natural Skincare

Choosing natural skincare over synthetic products can have numerous benefits, particularly for those mindful of what they put on their skin and how it affects their overall health and the environment.

Fewer Chemicals and Preservatives: One of the primary advantages of natural skincare is that it typically contains fewer chemicals and preservatives than conventional products. Many store-bought skincare items contain synthetic fragrances, parabens, sulfates, and other additives that can irritate the skin or lead to long-term health concerns. Natural skincare, on the other hand, uses ingredients derived from plants, fruits, and other natural sources, which are less likely to cause irritation and more likely to provide gentle, nurturing care for your skin.

Better for Sensitive Skin: If you have sensitive skin, you know how challenging it can be to find products that don't cause redness, dryness, or breakouts. Natural ingredients are more soothing and less likely to trigger adverse reactions. Aloe vera, chamomile, and honey are known for their calming properties, making them ideal for sensitive skin. You can enjoy the benefits of a more balanced, irritation-free complexion by choosing natural skincare.

Environmentally Friendly: Natural skincare is beneficial for your skin and the environment. Many synthetic skincare products contain microplastics, artificial ingredients, and other compounds that can harm the environment when washed down the drain. Natural ingredients are biodegradable and sourced from renewable resources, making them a more sustainable choice. Additionally, many DIY skincare enthusiasts prefer eco-friendly packaging, reducing their environmental footprint.

Essential Ingredients for DIY Skincare

Creating your skincare products at home can be a fun and rewarding experience. It lets you know what's going into your skincare routine and allows you to customize products to meet your specific needs. Here are some essential natural ingredients that are used in DIY skincare recipes:

Coconut Oil: Moisturizing and Antibacterial Coconut oil is a versatile ingredient that's beloved for its deep moisturizing properties. It's rich in fatty acids, which help to hydrate and nourish the skin, leaving it soft and supple. Coconut oil also has natural antibacterial and antifungal properties, making it an excellent choice for those prone to breakouts or skin infections. You can use it as a stand-alone moisturizer, makeup remover, or as a base for DIY skincare products.

Honey: Antioxidant and Anti-Inflammatory Honey is another powerhouse ingredient in natural skincare. It's packed with antioxidants that help protect the skin from free radical damage, and its natural anti-inflammatory properties can soothe irritated skin. Honey is also a humectant, which helps retain moisture in the skin, making it ideal for hydrating dry or mature skin. Organic honey is best for skincare, as it contains more beneficial enzymes and nutrients.

Aloe Vera: Soothing and Hydrating Aloe vera is well-known for its soothing and healing properties, making it a go-to ingredient for calming irritated or sunburned skin. It's also highly hydrating, providing moisture without leaving a greasy residue. Aloe vera gel can be used directly on the skin or mixed into other skincare recipes to enhance their soothing effects. It's particularly beneficial for those with sensitive or inflamed skin.

DIY Skincare Recipes

Ready to start crafting your skincare products? Here are a few simple and practical DIY recipes you can make with natural ingredients in your kitchen.

Homemade Face Masks: Honey and Avocado Mask This hydrating and nourishing face mask is perfect for dry or mature skin.

Ingredients:

- 1 tablespoon raw honey
- 1/2 ripe avocado
- 1 tablespoon plain yogurt (optional, for added moisture)

Instructions:

1 Mash the avocado in a small bowl until smooth.

2 Add the honey and yogurt (if using), and mix until well combined.

3 Apply the mask to clean skin, avoiding the eye area.

4 Leave the mask on for 15-20 minutes, then rinse off with warm water.

5 Follow with your usual moisturizer.

Natural Exfoliating Scrubs: Sugar and Olive Oil Scrub This simple scrub will leave your skin feeling soft, smooth, and rejuvenated.

Ingredients:

- 1/2 cup granulated sugar (brown or white)
- 1/4 cup olive oil
- 1 tablespoon honey
- A few drops of your favorite essential oil (optional, for fragrance)

Instructions:

1 Combine the sugar, olive oil, and honey in a bowl, stirring until well mixed.

2 Add a few drops of essential oil if you want a pleasant scent.

3 Gently massage the scrub onto damp skin in circular motions, focusing on elbows, knees, and feet.

4 Rinse off with warm water and pat your skin dry.

5 Use this scrub once or twice a week for best results.

Simple Moisturizers: Shea Butter and Essential Oils This rich moisturizer is perfect for keeping your skin soft and hydrated.

Ingredients:

• 1/2 cup shea butter

• 1/4 cup coconut oil

• 1/4 cup jojoba oil or almond oil

• 10-15 drops of your favorite essential oil (e.g., lavender, rose, or frankincense)

Instructions:

1 Melt the shea butter and coconut oil together in a double boiler or microwave.

2 Once melted, remove from heat and stir in the jojoba or almond oil.

3 Add the essential oil drops and mix well.

4 Pour the mixture into a clean, airtight container and let it cool until solid.

5 Apply a small amount to your skin as needed, particularly after bathing.

Skin Care Routine Tips

Now that you have some wonderful DIY skincare recipes, it's essential to incorporate them into a consistent skincare routine that suits your skin type and lifestyle. Here are a few tips to help you establish a natural skincare routine that works for you:

Morning and Evening Skincare Routines: A good skincare routine typically includes morning and evening steps. In the morning, focus on cleansing, moisturizing, and protecting your skin with a natural sunscreen. In the evening, cleanse your skin to remove makeup and impurities, follow with a nourishing face mask or serum, and finish with a rich moisturizer to hydrate your skin overnight. Consistency is vital—by following these steps daily, you'll help your skin stay healthy and radiant.

Importance of Patch Testing New Products: Whenever you introduce a new skincare product—especially a DIY one—it's crucial to do a patch test first. Apply a small amount of the product to an inconspicuous area of your skin, like the inside of your wrist, and wait 24 hours to see if there's any reaction. This simple step can help prevent potential allergic reactions or irritation, ensuring your new skincare routine is safe and effective for your skin type.

Tips for Consistent Skincare Habits: Sticking to a skincare routine can sometimes be challenging, but it's easier when you make it a habit. Set aside time each morning and evening for your skincare routine, and keep your products organized and easily accessible. You might also want to create a relaxing environment—light a candle, play soft music, or turn your routine into a calming ritual you look forward to daily. The more enjoyable you make the experience, the more likely you will stick with it.

By embracing natural skincare, you're taking care of your skin and consciously choosing to use safe, gentle, and environmentally friendly products. With these DIY recipes and tips, you can create a personalized skincare routine that nourishes your skin, boosts your confidence, and enhances your natural beauty as you age.

Balancing Hormones Naturally: Diet and Lifestyle Tips

As women age, hormonal changes can significantly impact health and well-being. These fluctuations, particularly during and after menopause, can lead to a variety of symptoms that affect both physical and emotional health. While these changes are a natural part of aging, there are many ways to support your body through this transition, such as diet, lifestyle adjustments, and natural remedies to help maintain hormonal balance and improve overall quality of life.

Understanding Hormones and Aging

Hormones are the body's chemical messengers, crucial in regulating many processes, from metabolism and energy levels to mood and reproductive health. As women age, particularly during the transition into menopause, hormonal levels fluctuate and eventually decline, leading to a variety of changes in the body.

Menopause and Hormonal Fluctuations: Menopause marks the end of a woman's reproductive years, defined as the cessation of menstrual periods for 12 consecutive months. This transition typically occurs between the ages of 45 and 55 but can vary widely. During menopause, levels of estrogen and progesterone—two critical hormones in the female body—decline significantly. These hormonal shifts can lead to a range of symptoms, including hot flashes, night sweats, mood swings, and changes in skin and hair.

Symptoms of Hormonal Imbalance: In addition to the natural changes that occur during menopause, other factors such as diet, stress, and lifestyle can contribute to hormonal imbalances. Symptoms of hormonal imbalance may include fatigue, weight gain, difficulty sleeping, decreased libido, and irregular menstrual cycles in the years leading up to menopause. These symptoms can be challenging, but by understanding the role of hormones and making targeted adjustments, it's possible to alleviate many of these issues and support a smoother transition through this stage of life.

Dietary Adjustments for Hormonal Balance

Your diet plays a vital role in maintaining hormonal balance. Certain foods can help regulate hormone levels and alleviate symptoms associated with hormonal fluctuations. Here are some dietary tips to help you achieve and maintain hormonal harmony:

Increasing Intake of Phytoestrogens: Phytoestrogens are naturally occurring plant compounds that mimic the effects of estrogen in the body. Including foods rich in phytoestrogens can help balance hormone levels, particularly during menopause. Flaxseeds, soy products (like tofu and tempeh), and legumes are excellent sources of phytoestrogens. For example, adding ground flaxseeds to your morning smoothie or incorporating tofu into your meals can provide your body with these beneficial compounds, helping to ease symptoms like hot flashes and mood swings.

Reducing Sugar and Refined Carbs: High sugar intake and refined carbohydrates can disrupt hormonal balance by causing spikes in blood sugar and insulin levels. This leads to increased production of androgens (male hormones) and exacerbates symptoms of hormonal imbalance. Reducing your sugary snacks, white bread, and pasta intake and focusing on whole grains, vegetables, and lean proteins can help stabilize blood sugar levels and support overall hormonal health.

Incorporating Healthy Fats: Healthy fats are essential for hormone production and overall health. Fats from sources like avocados, nuts, seeds, and oily fish (such as salmon) provide the building blocks your body needs to produce hormones. Omega-3 fatty acids, found in fish, flaxseeds, and chia seeds, are particularly beneficial for reducing inflammation and supporting heart and brain health, which are important considerations during menopause.

Lifestyle Changes for Hormonal Health

Critical lifestyle changes, in addition to dietary adjustments, can significantly impact hormonal balance and help manage the symptoms of aging.

Regular Physical Activity: Exercise is one of the most effective ways to balance hormones naturally. Regular physical activity helps regulate insulin levels, reduce stress hormones like cortisol, and boost endorphins, which improve mood and overall well-being. Aim for a mix of cardiovascular exercises, strength training, and flexibility exercises like yoga or Pilates. Daily walking can profoundly affect your hormonal health and help mitigate symptoms such as weight gain, fatigue, and mood swings.

Stress Management Techniques: Chronic stress is a significant contributor to hormonal imbalance. When you're stressed, your body produces more cortisol, a hormone that, in excess, can interfere with other hormones, leading to weight gain, sleep disturbances, and mood swings. Incorporating stress management techniques like meditation, deep breathing exercises, or yoga into your daily routine can help reduce cortisol levels and promote hormonal balance. Taking time for self-care, whether through a relaxing bath, a hobby you enjoy, or simply spending time in nature, is also crucial for managing stress and supporting your overall health.

Adequate Sleep and Sleep Hygiene: Quality sleep is essential for maintaining hormonal balance, yet many women experience sleep disturbances during menopause. Establishing good sleep hygiene can help improve the quality of your sleep, including maintaining a regular sleep schedule, creating a calming bedtime routine, and ensuring your sleep environment is comfortable and free of distractions. Reducing screen time before bed, limiting caffeine intake in the afternoon, and practicing relaxation techniques can all contribute to better sleep, supporting overall hormonal health.

Herbal Remedies

In addition to diet and lifestyle changes, certain herbs have traditionally supported hormonal balance and alleviated symptoms of menopause and hormonal fluctuations. Here are a few that you might consider incorporating into your routine:

Black Cohosh for Menopausal Symptoms: Black cohosh is a popular herbal remedy for alleviating menopausal symptoms, scorching hot flashes and night sweats. It has been used for centuries in traditional medicine and mimics the effects of estrogen in the body. While research on its effectiveness is inconclusive, many women find relief from menopausal symptoms when using black cohosh supplements. It's essential to consult with a healthcare provider before starting any new supplement, especially if you have any underlying health conditions.

Maca Root for Energy and Libido: Maca root, a plant native to the Andes, is often used to boost energy, stamina, and libido. It supports hormonal balance by nourishing the endocrine system, which regulates hormone production. Maca can be taken in powder form, added to smoothies, or as a supplement. Some women find that maca helps alleviate fatigue, improve mood, and enhance sexual well-being, making it a valuable addition to a natural approach to hormone health.

Vitex (Chasteberry) for Menstrual Regulation: Vitex, also known as chasteberry, is a herb commonly used to regulate menstrual cycles and alleviate symptoms of premenstrual syndrome (PMS). It influences the pituitary gland, which controls the release of hormones in the body. Vitex can be particularly beneficial for women in the perimenopausal stage who are experiencing irregular periods or PMS symptoms. As with any herbal remedy, it's essential to consult with a healthcare provider to ensure it's appropriate for your individual needs.

Balancing hormones naturally through diet, lifestyle, and herbal remedies can significantly improve your quality of life as you age. By making thoughtful adjustments to your diet, incorporating regular exercise, managing stress, and exploring natural supplements, you can support your body through the hormonal changes of aging with grace and vitality. Remember, small, consistent changes can significantly improve your feelings, helping you embrace this stage of life with confidence and energy.

Anti-Inflammatory Foods: Fighting Joint Pain with Diet

As we age, our bodies often face the cumulative effects of years of wear and tear, and one of the most common issues that can arise is joint pain. Chronic inflammation significantly contributes to joint pain and other age-related health problems. Fortunately, diet is influential in reducing inflammation, alleviating joint pain, and supporting overall health. This section will explore the relationship between inflammation and aging, introduce anti-inflammatory foods, and provide practical tips for incorporating these foods into daily meals.

The Role of Inflammation in Aging

Inflammation is a natural response of the immune system to injury or infection. While acute inflammation is necessary for healing, chronic inflammation can lead to various health issues, particularly as we age.

Link Between Inflammation and Arthritis: Chronic inflammation is linked to developing arthritis, including osteoarthritis and rheumatoid arthritis. Osteoarthritis occurs when the protective cartilage that cushions the ends of your bones wears down over time, leading to pain, swelling, and reduced joint mobility. In contrast, rheumatoid arthritis is an autoimmune disorder where the immune system attacks the body's tissues, causing joint inflammation and pain. Chronic inflammation exacerbates these conditions, increasing joint pain and stiffness (Giugliano, Ceriello, & Esposito, 2006).

Impact on Overall Health: Beyond joint pain, chronic inflammation is a significant risk factor for several age-related diseases, including cardiovascular disease, diabetes, and certain types of cancer (Ridker & Luscher, 2014). By managing inflammation through diet and lifestyle, you can reduce joint pain, improve your overall health, and extend your lifespan.

Top Anti-Inflammatory Foods

Incorporating anti-inflammatory foods into your diet is one of the most effective ways to combat chronic inflammation and support joint health. Here are some of the top foods known for their anti-inflammatory properties:

Turmeric: Curcumin's Anti-Inflammatory Properties Turmeric is a vibrant yellow spice commonly used in Indian cuisine. It is renowned for its powerful anti-inflammatory effects, primarily due to a compound called curcumin. Curcumin reduces inflammation by inhibiting molecules that play a role in the inflammatory process (Gupta, Patchva, & Aggarwal, 2013). Adding turmeric to your diet can be as simple as incorporating it into soups, stews, or smoothies. For enhanced absorption, pair turmeric with black pepper, which contains piperine, which increases curcumin's bioavailability (Rao & Waseem, 2013).

Fatty Fish: Omega-3 Fatty Acids Fatty fish such as salmon, mackerel, and sardines are rich in omega-3 fatty acids, essential fats with potent anti-inflammatory properties. Omega-3s help reduce the production of inflammatory molecules and decrease the severity of symptoms in conditions like rheumatoid arthritis (Mozaffarian & Wu, 2012). Aim to include fatty fish in your diet at least twice weekly to reap the anti-inflammatory benefits. If you're not a fan of fish, omega-3 supplements, such as fish or algae oil, can also be effective (Calder, 2010).

Berries: Antioxidants and Anti-Inflammatory Effects Berries, including blueberries, strawberries, and raspberries, are packed with antioxidants, particularly anthocyanins, which have potent anti-inflammatory effects. These antioxidants help neutralize free radicals in the body, reducing inflammation and protecting against cellular damage (Miller & Shukitt-Hale, 2012). Berries are also high in fiber and low in calories, making them a nutritious addition to your diet. Enjoy them as a snack, add them to your morning oatmeal, or blend them into smoothies for a delicious, anti-inflammatory boost.

Green Tea: Polyphenols and Antioxidants Green tea is another excellent addition to an anti-inflammatory diet thanks to its high content of polyphenols, particularly epigallocatechin gallate (EGCG). EGCG is a powerful antioxidant that reduces inflammation and protects against chronic diseases (Johnson, Mukhtar, & Ahmad, 2010). Drinking green tea regularly can help lower inflammation levels, making it a soothing and healthful beverage choice. Aim for two to three cups a day to maximize its benefits.

Meal Planning for an Anti-Inflammatory Diet

Planning your meals around anti-inflammatory foods can make incorporating these beneficial ingredients into your diet easier. Here are some tips to help you get started:

Weekly Meal Plans with Recipes: A weekly meal plan focusing on anti-inflammatory foods can simplify your shopping and cooking process. Select essential breakfast, lunch, and dinner recipes with anti-inflammatory ingredients like fatty fish, berries, leafy greens, and whole grains. For example, you might plan a week that provides turmeric-spiced grilled salmon, quinoa, kale salad, and a berry-packed smoothie for breakfast. Rotating different recipes each week can help keep your meals exciting and nutritionally balanced.

Grocery Shopping Lists: Once you've planned your meals, create a grocery list with all the necessary ingredients. Focus on whole foods like fresh fruits and vegetables, lean proteins, healthy fats, and whole grains. Avoid processed foods, which often contain added sugars, unhealthy fats, and preservatives that can contribute to inflammation (O'Keefe, Gheewala, & O'Keefe, 2008). Shopping with a list can help you stay organized and ensure you have everything you need to prepare anti-inflammatory meals.

Batch Cooking and Meal Prep Tips: Batch cooking and meal prep can save you time and make it easier to stick to your anti-inflammatory diet throughout the week. Dedicate a few hours on the weekend to cook larger portions of essential components like grains, proteins, and roasted vegetables. Store them in the fridge or freezer to quickly assemble meals during busy weekdays. Preparing ingredients like chopping vegetables or marinating fish ahead of time can also streamline your cooking process, making it easier to enjoy healthy, homemade meals every day.

Success Stories

Hearing from others who have experienced the benefits of an anti-inflammatory diet can be incredibly motivating. Here are a few testimonials from women who have successfully reduced joint pain and improved their health by embracing an anti-inflammatory approach:

Personal Anecdotes on Decreased Pain and Increased Mobility:

- **Karen, 65:** "I've struggled with arthritis for years, and it was getting to the point where I could barely walk without pain. After reading about the benefits of an anti-inflammatory diet, I decided to try it. I started incorporating more turmeric and fatty fish into my meals and cut back on processed foods. Within a few months, I noticed a significant reduction in my joint pain. I can now go on walks again, and I feel like I've regained a sense of freedom and mobility I thought I had lost forever."

- **Linda, 58:** "When I hit menopause, I began experiencing joint pain and stiffness that I hadn't dealt with before. My doctor recommended an anti-inflammatory diet, so I added more berries, leafy greens, and green tea to my routine. The changes didn't happen overnight, but after a few months, I realized I was waking up without the usual aches and pains. My joint pain has decreased, and I feel more energized and less sluggish overall."

These stories highlight an anti-inflammatory diet's powerful impact on health and quality of life. By making mindful food choices and incorporating anti-inflammatory ingredients into one's meals, one can take control of one's health, reduce joint pain, and enjoy a more active, pain-free lifestyle.

Gut Health: The Key to Overall Wellness

Gut health is a cornerstone of overall wellness, with growing research highlighting its influence on various aspects of physical and mental health. A well-functioning gut is crucial for effective digestion, nutrient absorption, immune function, and mental well-being. In this section, we will explore the importance of gut health, the role of probiotics and prebiotics, dietary tips for maintaining a healthy gut, and daily practices that can support gut health.

Importance of Gut Health

The gut plays a pivotal role in maintaining overall health, and disruptions in gut function can lead to a wide range of health issues.

Role in Digestion and Nutrient Absorption: The primary function of the gut is to break down the food we eat, enabling the absorption of essential nutrients like vitamins, minerals, and amino acids. A healthy gut ensures this process occurs efficiently, supporting overall bodily functions. When gut health is compromised, it can result in poor nutrient absorption, leading to deficiencies and various health problems (Rao & Samak, 2012).

Connection to Immune Health and Mental Well-Being: Approximately 70% of the immune system resides in the gut, making it a critical player in immune defense (Mowat & Agace, 2014). The gut microbiota, which consists of trillions of microorganisms, helps regulate immune responses and protect against pathogens. Moreover, the gut-brain axis —a bidirectional communication network between the gut and brain —links gut health to mental well-being. Disruptions in gut microbiota can influence mood and cognitive function, contributing to conditions such as anxiety and depression (Carabotti et al., 2015).

Probiotics and Prebiotics

Include probiotics and prebiotics in your diet to maintain a healthy gut. These elements work synergistically to support a balanced gut microbiome.

Sources of Probiotics: Probiotics are live beneficial bacteria that help maintain a healthy gut by outcompeting harmful bacteria and promoting digestive health. Familiar sources of probiotics include:

- **Yogurt:** Contains live cultures of beneficial bacteria such as *Lactobacillus* and *Bifidobacterium* (McFarland, 2015).
- **Kefir:** A fermented milk drink rich in various probiotic strains that support gut health (Farnworth, 2005).
- **Sauerkraut and Kimchi:** Fermented cabbage dishes that are rich in probiotics and also provide dietary fiber, which supports digestion (Marco et al., 2017).

Sources of Prebiotics: Prebiotics are non-digestible fibers that serve as food for beneficial gut bacteria, helping them thrive. Critical sources of prebiotics include:

- **Garlic:** Contains inulin, a fiber that promotes the growth of beneficial *Bifidobacteria* in the gut (Roberfroid, 2007).
- **Onions:** Rich in fructooligosaccharides (FOS), a prebiotic fiber that supports gut health (Slavin, 2013).
- **Bananas:** Particularly when slightly under-ripe, bananas are a good source of resistant starch, which acts as a prebiotic (Slavin, 2013).

Dietary Tips for a Healthy Gut

Supporting gut health through diet is essential for maintaining overall wellness. Here are some dietary recommendations that can help promote a healthy gut.

High-Fiber Foods: Fiber is crucial for gut health as it aids digestion and fuels beneficial gut bacteria. Foods high in fiber include whole grains like oats and barley and legumes such as beans and lentils. A high-fiber diet helps regulate bowel movements, reduces the risk of digestive disorders, and supports a diverse gut microbiome (Slavin, 2013).

Fermented Foods for Probiotics: Besides the probiotic-rich foods mentioned earlier, fermented foods such as miso, tempeh, and pickles can contribute to gut health. These foods enhance the diversity of your gut microbiota and improve digestion and immune function (Marco et al., 2017).

Reducing Processed Foods and Sugars: Processed foods and refined sugars can disrupt the balance of bacteria in the gut, leading to increased inflammation and digestive issues. These foods are often low in fiber and high in additives that can harm gut health. Reducing processed foods and sugar intake and focusing on whole, nutrient-dense foods can help maintain a healthy gut environment (Vogt et al., 2017).

Gut Health Practices

Beyond diet, certain daily practices can further support gut health and contribute to overall well-being.

Staying Hydrated: Hydration is essential for digestion, as water helps break down food and facilitates nutrient absorption. It also keeps the digestive tract lubricated, preventing constipation and promoting regular bowel movements. Drinking plenty of water throughout the day is a simple yet effective way to support gut health (Popkin et al., 2010).

Regular Physical Activity: Exercise has numerous benefits for gut health, including promoting regular bowel movements and reducing the risk of constipation. Physical activity also supports a healthy gut microbiome by enhancing the diversity of beneficial bacteria and reducing inflammation (Mach & Fuster-Botella, 2017). Aim for regular exercise, such as walking, swimming, or yoga, to support your digestive health.

Mindful Eating Habits: Mindful eating involves paying attention to the eating experience, chewing food thoroughly, and eating slowly. This practice can improve digestion by allowing your body to break down and absorb nutrients properly. Additionally, mindful eating can help prevent overeating and reduce stress, essential for maintaining a healthy gut (Miller et al., 2012).

Maintaining gut health is vital to overall wellness. By incorporating probiotics and prebiotics into your diet, focusing on high-fiber and fermented foods, and adopting healthy lifestyle practices, you can support a healthy gut and, in turn, improve your overall health. A healthy gut enhances digestion and nutrient absorption and promotes immune function and mental well-being, making it essential to a healthy, balanced life.

3

HOLISTIC HEALTH AND WELLNESS

Yoga for All Ages: Gentle Poses for Strength and Flexibility

Yoga is an ancient practice that offers many physical and mental health benefits, making it particularly valuable for older adults. Maintaining strength, flexibility, and balance becomes increasingly important as we age, and yoga provides a gentle yet effective way to achieve these goals. In this chapter, we will explore the benefits of yoga for aging, introduce gentle yoga poses suitable for all ages, offer tips on creating a consistent yoga practice, and share success stories of individuals who have incorporated yoga into their daily routines.

Benefits of Yoga for Aging

Yoga is a low-impact exercise accessible to people of all ages and fitness levels. For older adults, yoga offers specific benefits that can help maintain physical health and improve quality of life.

Improved Flexibility and Balance: One of the primary benefits of yoga is its ability to improve flexibility and balance, which are essential for preventing falls and maintaining mobility as we age. Regular yoga stretches and poses help to lengthen muscles and increase the range of motion in the joints, making everyday movements more manageable and fluid (Cowan & Adams, 2020). Additionally, yoga's focus on balance through poses like Tree Pose can enhance stability, reducing the risk of falls (Youkhana et al., 2016).

Enhanced Muscle Strength: Yoga is also an effective way to build and maintain muscle strength, which is crucial for supporting bone health and preventing age-related muscle loss (osteoporosis). Poses that involve weight-bearing, such as Downward Dog and Warrior poses, engage multiple muscle groups, promoting overall strength and endurance. Unlike traditional strength training, yoga builds muscle strength in a balanced way, reducing the risk of injury and improving posture (Bower & Sternlicht, 2014).

Better Joint Health: For those suffering from joint pain or arthritis, yoga can be a gentle yet powerful tool for improving joint health. The slow, controlled movements in yoga help lubricate the joints, increase circulation, and reduce stiffness. Poses that focus on joint mobility, such as Cat-Cow Pose, can help maintain joint flexibility and alleviate pain associated with arthritis (Kolasinski et al., 2020).

Reduced Stress and Anxiety: Besides its physical benefits, yoga is well-known for its ability to reduce stress and anxiety. Deep, mindful breathing, combined with gentle movement, activates the parasympathetic nervous system, promoting relaxation and reducing the production of stress hormones like cortisol (Streeter et al., 2012). Yoga offers a calming practice that supports mental well-being for older adults who may face increased stress due to health concerns or life transitions.

Gentle Yoga Poses

For those new to yoga or seeking a gentle practice, the following poses are excellent for improving strength, flexibility, and relaxation. These poses are accessible to individuals of all ages and can be modified to suit different ability levels.

Cat-Cow Pose (Marjaryasana-Bitilasana) for Spine Flexibility: Cat-Cow Pose is a dynamic sequence that promotes spine flexibility and warms back muscles.

- **Instructions:**

1 Start on your hands and knees in a tabletop position, with your wrists aligned under your shoulders and your knees under your hips.

2 Inhale as you arch your back, dropping your belly towards the mat and lifting your head and tailbone towards the ceiling (Cow Pose).

3 Exhale as you round your back, tucking your chin to your chest and drawing your belly towards your spine (Cat Pose).

4 Continue flowing between these two poses with each breath, moving slowly and gently.

Cat-Cow Pose is particularly beneficial for older adults as it increases spinal flexibility and improves posture, helping to alleviate back pain (Cramer et al., 2013).

Child's Pose (Balasana) for Relaxation and Stretching: Child's Pose is a restful pose that provides a gentle stretch to the back, hips, and thighs, promoting relaxation.

- **Instructions:**

1 Begin kneeling with your big toes touching and your knees spread apart.

2 Sit back on your heels and extend your arms forward, lowering your torso between your thighs.

3 Rest your forehead on the mat and breathe deeply, allowing your body to relax and release tension.

4 Hold the pose for several breaths or as long as it feels comfortable.

Child's pose is a calming pose that helps to stretch the lower back and hips, making it ideal for those who experience tension or stiffness in these areas (Field, 2016).

Seated Forward Bend (Paschimottanasana) for Hamstring Flexibility: Seated Forward Bend is a gentle stretch that targets the hamstrings and lower back, promoting flexibility and relaxation.

- **Instructions:**

1 Sit on the floor with your legs extended straight in front of you and your spine tall.

2 Inhale as you reach your arms overhead, lengthening your spine.

3 Exhale as you hinge at your hips, reaching forward towards your feet while keeping your back straight.

4 Depending on your flexibility, hold onto your shins, ankles, or feet, and breathe deeply.

5 Stay in the pose for several breaths, allowing your body to relax into the stretch.

Seated Forward Bend helps to release tension in the hamstrings and lower back, which can be particularly beneficial for older adults who may experience tightness in these areas (Sherman et al., 2011).

Bridge Pose (Setu Bandhasana) for Strengthening the Back and Glutes: Bridge Pose is a gentle backbend that strengthens the back muscles, glutes, and hamstrings while opening the chest and improving posture.

- **Instructions:**

1 Lie on your back with your knees bent and feet flat on the floor, hip-width apart.

2 Place your arms by your sides with your palms facing down.

3 Inhale as you press into your feet and lift your hips towards the ceiling, engaging your glutes and lower back.

4 Hold the pose for a few breaths, keeping your thighs parallel and your chest open.

5 Exhale as you slowly lower your hips back to the floor.

Bridge Pose is an excellent pose for building strength in the back and glutes, essential for maintaining mobility and stability as we age (Lauche et al., 2016).

Meditation and Mindfulness: Techniques for Inner Peace

Finding moments of inner peace can be challenging in our fast-paced world, yet it is essential for maintaining overall well-being. Meditation and mindfulness practices offer powerful tools for cultivating calm, improving mental clarity, and enhancing emotional resilience. This section will explore the benefits of meditation and mindfulness, introduce simple meditation techniques, suggest daily mindfulness practices, and offer guidance on creating a peaceful meditation space at home.

Introduction to Meditation

Meditation and mindfulness are ancient practices that have gained significant attention recently for their profound benefits on mental and emotional health. While these practices can take many forms, they generally involve focusing the mind and cultivating awareness in the present moment.

Reducing Stress and Anxiety: One of the most well-documented benefits of meditation is its ability to reduce stress and anxiety. By promoting relaxation and encouraging a shift in perspective, meditation helps lower the production of stress hormones like cortisol (Hoge et al., 2013). This stress reduction improves mental well-being and positively impacts physical health, reducing the risk of stress-related conditions such as hypertension and heart disease (Goyal et al., 2014).

Improving Focus and Concentration: Meditation is also known for enhancing focus and concentration. Regular practice helps train the mind to stay attentive and reduce distractions, improving cognitive performance and productivity (Zeidan et al., 2010). Whether used for personal development or professional tasks, meditation provides a mental workout that strengthens the brain's ability to concentrate.

Enhancing Emotional Well-Being: Beyond its cognitive benefits, meditation promotes self-awareness and emotional regulation. Through practices such as mindfulness, individuals learn to observe their thoughts and feelings without judgment, leading to a greater sense of emotional balance and resilience (Keng, Smoski, & Robins, 2011). Meditation also increases positive emotions and reduces symptoms of depression (Hofmann et al., 2010).

Simple Meditation Techniques

For those new to meditation or looking to deepen their practice, the following techniques offer a simple and accessible way to begin.

Breath-Focused Meditation: Breath-focused meditation is one of the most fundamental and widely practiced forms of meditation. It involves focusing on the breath to anchor the mind in the present moment.

• **Instructions:**

1 Find a comfortable position on a cushion or a chair, with your spine straight and your hands resting on your lap.

2 Close your eyes and take a few deep breaths, then allow your breathing to settle into a natural rhythm.

3 Focus on the sensation of your breath as it enters and leaves your nostrils or the rise and fall of your chest.

4 If your mind wanders, gently bring your focus back to your breath without judgment.

5 Continue this practice for 5 to 10 minutes, gradually increasing the duration as you become more comfortable with the technique.

Breath-focused meditation effectively calms the mind and reduces stress, making it a great starting point for beginners (Zeidan et al., 2010).

Body Scan Meditation: Body scan meditation involves bringing attention to different body parts, promoting relaxation and awareness of physical sensations.

• **Instructions:**

1 Lie on your back or sit comfortably in a chair, with your hands resting at your sides or lap.

2 Close your eyes and take a few deep breaths to relax.

3 Begin by focusing on your toes and noticing any sensations or tension.

4 Gradually move your attention up through your body—your feet, legs, abdomen, chest, arms, and finally, your head—pausing at each area to observe how it feels.

5 If you notice any tension, release it with each exhale.

6 Once you've scanned your entire body, take a moment to observe how you feel before gently bringing your awareness back to the present.

Body scan meditation is particularly beneficial for those who experience physical tension or discomfort, as it encourages deep relaxation and body awareness (Kabat-Zinn, 2005).

Loving-Kindness Meditation: Loving-kindness meditation (also known as Metta meditation) focuses on cultivating compassion and kindness towards oneself and others.

• **Instructions:**

1 Sit comfortably and close your eyes, taking a few deep breaths to settle in.

2 Begin by silently repeating well-wishing phrases to yourself, such as "May I be happy, may I be healthy, may I be safe, may I live with ease."

3 After a few minutes, extend these wishes to others—first to someone you love, then to a neutral person, and finally to someone you have difficulty with.

4 As you offer these phrases, try to feel the kindness and compassion behind the words genuinely.

5 Conclude by extending loving-kindness to all beings everywhere.

Loving-kindness meditation is a powerful practice for enhancing emotional well-being, fostering empathy, and reducing anger or resentment (Hofmann et al., 2011).

Mindfulness Practices

In addition to formal meditation, incorporating mindfulness into daily activities can enhance overall well-being and bring greater awareness to everyday life.

Mindful Breathing Exercises: Mindful breathing can be practiced anywhere, any time, making it a versatile tool for managing stress and staying present.

• **Instructions:**

1 Take a moment to pause, wherever you are.

2 Focus on your breath, noticing the sensation of the air entering and leaving your body.

3 If your mind wanders, gently guide it back to the rhythm of your breath.

4 Practice this for a few minutes whenever you need to center yourself.

Mindful breathing is an excellent way to quickly reduce stress and return to the present moment, especially during busy or challenging times (Brown & Ryan, 2003).

Mindful Eating Practices: Mindful eating involves paying full attention to the eating experience, from the taste and texture of the food to the sensations in your body.

• **Instructions:**

1 Begin by taking a few deep breaths to calm your mind before eating.

2 Eat slowly, savoring each bite, and pay attention to your food's flavors, textures, and aromas.

3 Notice how your body feels as you eat—whether you're hungry, satisfied, or full.

4 Avoid distractions like television or smartphones, allowing yourself to experience the act of eating fully.

Mindful eating can help improve digestion, promote healthier eating habits, and enhance the enjoyment of food (Kristeller & Wolever, 2011).

Walking Meditation: Walking meditation is a form of mindfulness practice that focuses on walking, bringing awareness to each step and the sensations in your body.

• **Instructions:**

1 Find a quiet place where you can walk without distractions.

2 Begin strolling, paying attention to the movement of your feet and legs.

3 Notice the sensation of your feet touching the ground, your muscles' movement, and your breath's rhythm.

4 If your mind wanders, gently bring your attention back to the physical sensations of walking.

5 Continue this practice for several minutes, gradually increasing the duration as you become more comfortable.

Walking meditation is a great way to integrate mindfulness into your daily routine, especially if you enjoy being outdoors (Teasdale et al., 2000).

Creating a Meditation Space

Creating a dedicated meditation space at home can help establish a consistent practice and provide a peaceful environment for relaxation and reflection.

Choosing a Quiet, Comfortable Spot: Select a quiet area in your home where you can practice meditation without interruptions. This place could be a corner of a room, a spare bedroom, or even a section of your living room. The key is to choose a space where you feel comfortable and can relax fully (Siegel, 2010).

Using Cushions and Mats: Comfort is essential for meditation, especially if you plan to sit for extended periods. Invest in a meditation cushion (zafu) or a yoga mat to support your back and hips. You can also use a chair if sitting on the floor is uncomfortable (Goleman, 1996).

Incorporating Calming Elements: Enhance your meditation space with calming elements like candles, soft lighting, or soothing music. Adding a plant or a small fountain can also create a serene atmosphere. The goal is to create a space that invites relaxation and mindfulness (Kabat-Zinn, 2005).

Integrating meditation and mindfulness practices into daily life can cultivate inner peace, improve mental clarity, and enhance overall well-being. Whether you practice formal meditation or incorporate mindfulness into everyday activities, these techniques offer powerful tools for navigating the stresses of life with greater ease and resilience.

Herbal Remedies: Nature's Medicine Cabinet

Herbal remedies have been used for centuries to treat a variety of health conditions and to promote overall wellness. In recent years, there has been a resurgence of interest in herbal medicine as more people seek natural and holistic approaches to healthcare. This section will explore the benefits of herbal remedies, introduce some of the most common medicinal herbs, provide guidance on preparing herbal remedies at home, and discuss the importance of safety and proper dosage.

Introduction to Herbal Remedies

Herbal remedies offer a natural alternative or complement to conventional medical treatments, and they can be highly effective for managing a wide range of health issues.

Natural and Fewer Side Effects: One of the primary advantages of herbal remedies is that they are derived from natural sources and have fewer side effects than synthetic medications (Ekor, 2014). For example, chamomile, a popular herb for promoting relaxation and sleep, is generally well-tolerated and has minimal side effects when used appropriately (Srivastava, Shankar, & Gupta, 2010). This gentleness makes herbal remedies attractive for individuals seeking gentle, effective treatments with a lower risk of adverse reactions.

Complementary to Conventional Treatments: Herbal remedies can also be used alongside conventional treatments to enhance their effectiveness or alleviate side effects. For instance, ginger can reduce nausea, including nausea caused by chemotherapy (Ernst & Pittler, 2000). Ginger can provide additional relief when used with conventional anti-nausea medications, improving the overall treatment experience.

Cost-Effective: Another benefit of herbal remedies is their cost-effectiveness. Many medicinal herbs can be grown at home or purchased relatively cheaply, making them an accessible option for those seeking affordable healthcare solutions (Ekor, 2014). Additionally, preparing herbal remedies at home can further reduce costs while allowing individuals to customize treatments.

Common Herbs and Their Uses

Various herbs are used in herbal medicine, each with unique properties and health benefits. Below are some of the most common herbs and their medicinal uses.

Echinacea for Immune Support: Echinacea is a well-known herb often used to support the immune system, particularly during cold and flu season. Research suggests that echinacea can help reduce the duration and severity of colds by stimulating the body's natural defenses (Shah, Sander, & White, 2007). It is commonly taken as a tea, tincture, or supplement.

Chamomile for Relaxation and Sleep: Chamomile is widely used for its calming effects and is particularly popular as a remedy for insomnia and anxiety. The herb contains compounds like apigenin, which bind to receptors in the brain that promote relaxation (Srivastava et al., 2010). Chamomile tea is a simple and effective way to unwind before bed and improve sleep quality.

Ginger for Digestive Health: Ginger is a versatile herb with potent anti-inflammatory and antioxidant properties. It is especially effective for alleviating digestive issues such as nausea, bloating, and indigestion (Ernst & Pittler, 2000). Ginger can be consumed in various forms, including fresh, powdered, or as a tea.

Turmeric for Anti-Inflammatory Benefits: Turmeric, a bright yellow spice commonly used in Indian cuisine, is renowned for its powerful anti-inflammatory effects, primarily due to its active compound, curcumin. Studies have shown that turmeric can help reduce inflammation and pain, making it beneficial for arthritis (Gupta, Patchva, & Aggarwal, 2013). Turmeric can be added to foods, taken as a supplement, or used to make a healing tea.

Preparing Herbal Remedies at Home

Making herbal remedies at home is a rewarding and cost-effective way to support your health. Here are some simple recipes and instructions for preparing herbal teas, tinctures, and salves.

Herbal Teas: Herbal teas are one of the easiest ways to enjoy the benefits of medicinal herbs.

- **Chamomile Tea:**
  - Ingredients: 1 tablespoon of dried chamomile flowers, 1 cup of boiling water.
  - Instructions: Place the chamomile flowers in a teapot or mug. Pour boiling water over the flowers and steep for 5-10 minutes. Strain and enjoy before bedtime.
- **Peppermint Tea:**
  - Ingredients: 1 tablespoon of dried peppermint leaves, 1 cup of boiling water.
  - Instructions: Place the peppermint leaves in a teapot or mug.

Pour boiling water over the leaves and steep for 5-10 minutes. Strain and drink to soothe digestion.

Tinctures and Extracts: Tinctures are concentrated herbal extracts made by soaking herbs in alcohol or vinegar.

• **Elderberry Syrup:**

○ Ingredients: 1 cup of dried elderberries, 3 cups of water, 1 cup of honey.

○ Instructions: Combine elderberries and water in a saucepan and bring to a boil. Reduce heat and simmer for 30-45 minutes. Strain the mixture and discard the berries. Once cooled, stir in honey and store the syrup in a glass jar in the refrigerator. Take 1 tablespoon daily for immune support.

Salves and Balms: Herbal salves are soothing topical treatments made by infusing herbs in oil and thickening the mixture with beeswax.

• **Calendula Salve:**

○ Ingredients: 1 cup of dried calendula flowers, 1 cup of olive oil, 1/4 cup of beeswax.

○ Instructions: Infuse the calendula flowers in olive oil by placing them in a jar and covering them with oil. Let it sit for 2-4 weeks, shaking occasionally. Strain the oil and heat it in a double boiler with the beeswax until melted. Pour into a tin or jar and allow to cool. Use on dry or irritated skin.

Safety and Dosage

While herbal remedies offer many benefits, using them safely and understanding proper dosages is essential.

Consulting with a Healthcare Provider: Before starting any new herbal remedy, it is advisable to consult with a healthcare provider, especially if you are pregnant, breastfeeding, or have existing health conditions (Ekor, 2014). A healthcare provider can help ensure your chosen herbs are safe and appropriate for your needs.

Avoiding Interactions with Medications: Some herbs can interact with prescription medications, enhancing or reducing their effects. For example, St. John's Wort can interfere with the effectiveness of certain antidepressants (Greeson, Sanford, & Monti, 2001). Researching potential interactions and discussing them with your healthcare provider is crucial.

Following Recommended Dosages: Herbal remedies should be used in moderation, following recommended dosages to avoid potential side effects. Overuse of certain herbs, such as kava or comfrey, can lead to serious health issues (Teschke & Wolff, 2009). Always start with the lowest effective dose and adjust as needed based on your response.

By understanding the benefits of herbal remedies, learning to prepare them at home, and using them safely, you can harness the power of nature's medicine cabinet to support your health and well-being.

Aromatherapy: Using Essential Oils for Stress Relief

Aromatherapy is a holistic healing practice that utilizes essential oils to promote physical, mental, and emotional well-being. By harnessing the power of scent, aromatherapy can help reduce stress, improve sleep, and enhance overall mood. In this section, we will explore the benefits of aromatherapy, introduce some common essential oils used for stress relief, provide instructions on how to use essential oils, and share DIY recipes for creating your aromatherapy products.

Introduction to Aromatherapy

Aromatherapy involves using concentrated plant extracts, known as essential oils, which have therapeutic properties. These oils can be inhaled, applied to the skin, or used in baths to evoke a range of health benefits.

Reducing Stress and Anxiety: One of aromatherapy's primary benefits is its ability to reduce stress and anxiety. Essential oils like lavender and chamomile have calming effects on the nervous system, helping to lower cortisol levels and promote relaxation (Conrad & Adams, 2012). Inhaling the scent of these oils can trigger the brain's limbic system, which controls emotions, reducing stress and anxiety (Goel, Kim, & Lao, 2005).

Improving Sleep Quality: Aromatherapy is also widely used to enhance sleep quality. Essential oils such as lavender and valerian root promote restful sleep by calming the mind and body (Hwang & Shin, 2015). Diffusing these oils in the bedroom or applying them topically before bedtime can create a soothing environment that supports better sleep.

Enhancing Mood and Relaxation: Aromatherapy can enhance mood and relaxation, reduce stress, and improve sleep. Essential oils like bergamot and ylang-ylang are known for their uplifting properties, which can help alleviate depression and promote well-being (Hongratanaworakit, 2011). Incorporating these oils into your daily routine can help maintain emotional balance and foster a positive outlook.

Common Essential Oils

A variety of essential oils are used in aromatherapy for their stress-relieving properties. Here are some of the most popular ones:

Lavender for Relaxation: Lavender is one of the most well-known and versatile essential oils, particularly valued for its calming effects. Research has shown that lavender oil can reduce anxiety and promote relaxation, making it an excellent choice for stress relief and improving sleep (Conrad & Adams, 2012).

Peppermint for Mental Clarity: Peppermint oil is invigorating and refreshing, making it ideal for enhancing mental clarity and focus. Its cooling effect can also help relieve tension headaches and reduce feelings of fatigue (Moss, Hewitt, & Moss, 2012). Inhaling peppermint oil can boost alertness and improve cognitive performance, making it useful during mental exertion.

Eucalyptus for Respiratory Health: Eucalyptus oil is often used for its respiratory benefits, as it helps to clear the airways and ease breathing. Its refreshing scent can reduce stress and improve concentration while supporting respiratory health (Juergens et al., 2003). Eucalyptus oil is particularly beneficial during cold and flu season or when dealing with allergies.

Frankincense for Emotional Balance: Frankincense is known for its grounding and centering effects, making it a valuable oil for promoting emotional balance. It has been used for centuries in meditation and spiritual practices to enhance focus and tranquility (Woronuk et al., 2011). Frankincense oil can be diffused or applied topically to help manage stress and promote inner peace.

Methods of Use

Essential oils can be used in various ways, depending on your preferences and desired outcomes. Here are some methods of using essential oils for stress relief:

Diffusing Essential Oils: Diffusing is one of the most popular methods of using essential oils. A diffuser disperses the oils into the air, allowing you to inhale their therapeutic aromas.

• **Instructions:**

1 Fill your diffuser with water according to the manufacturer's instructions.

2 Add 5-10 drops of your chosen essential oil or a blend of oils.

3 Turn on the diffuser and enjoy the calming atmosphere it creates.

Diffusing essential oils can fill a room with a soothing scent that can help reduce stress and improve mood (Lee & Lee, 2014).

Topical Application with Carrier Oils: Essential oils can also be applied directly to the skin when diluted with a carrier oil, such as jojoba, coconut, or almond oil.

• **Instructions:**

1 Mix a few drops of essential oil with a carrier oil (approximately 1-2% dilution for adults).

2 Apply the mixture to pulse points, such as the wrists, temples, or the back of the neck.

3 Massage the oil into the skin and breathe deeply to absorb the benefits.

Topical application allows the oils to be absorbed into the bloodstream, where they can exert their calming effects (Tisserand & Young, 2013).

Aromatherapy Baths: Aromatherapy baths combine warm water's relaxing effects with essential oils' therapeutic properties.

• **Instructions:**

1 Fill your bathtub with warm water.

2 Add 5-10 drops of essential oil to a carrier or unscented bath salt, then add the mixture to the water.

3 Soak in the bath for 20-30 minutes, inhaling the calming aroma.

Aromatherapy baths are a fantastic way to unwind after a long day and can help reduce stress and promote relaxation (Cavanagh & Wilkinson, 2002).

DIY Aromatherapy Recipes

Creating your aromatherapy products at home is a simple and cost-effective way to enjoy the benefits of essential oils. Here are some easy DIY recipes for stress relief:

Calming Room Spray:

• **Ingredients:** 1 cup of distilled water, 1 tablespoon of witch hazel, 10 drops of lavender oil, 5 drops of bergamot oil.

• **Instructions:** Combine all ingredients in a spray bottle and shake well. Spritz the mixture around your home to create a calming atmosphere.

Relaxing Massage Oil:

• **Ingredients:** 2 tablespoons of almond oil, 5 drops of lavender oil, 3 drops of ylang-ylang oil.

• **Instructions:** Mix the oils in a small bottle. Use the oil for a relaxing massage, focusing on areas of tension like the shoulders and neck.

Stress-Relief Bath Salts:

• **Ingredients:** 1 cup of Epsom salts, 1/2 cup of baking soda, 10 drops of eucalyptus oil, 5 drops of peppermint oil.

• **Instructions:** Combine all ingredients in a jar and mix well. Add 1/4 cup of the mixture to your bathwater and soak to relieve stress and tension.

By incorporating aromatherapy into your daily routine, you can create a peaceful environment that supports mental and emotional well-being. Whether through diffusing essential oils, applying them topically, or enjoying an aromatherapy bath, these practices offer a natural and effective way to manage stress and promote relaxation.

Detoxing Your Life: Reducing Exposure to Toxins

In our modern world, we are surrounded by toxins that can negatively impact our health. From the products we use in our homes to the foods we consume, toxins can accumulate in our bodies, potentially leading to various health issues. This section will explore toxins, how they affect our health, and practical steps to reduce exposure through detoxifying your home, diet, and daily practices.

Understanding Toxins

Toxins are harmful substances that can come from various sources, both natural and human-made. These substances can disrupt bodily functions and contribute to chronic health problems.

Sources of Toxins: Toxins invade many aspects of daily life, including household products, food, and the environment. Everyday sources include cleaning products that contain harsh chemicals, processed foods with artificial additives, and environmental pollutants like pesticides and heavy metals (Landrigan, Fuller, & Acosta, 2018). Even seemingly innocuous items like plastic containers can release toxins such as bisphenol A (BPA) when heated, leaching into food or beverages (Vandenberg et al., 2007).

Impact on the Body: Exposure to toxins can have a wide range of effects on the body, including hormone disruption, immune suppression, and increased risk of chronic diseases. For example, endocrine-disrupting chemicals (EDCs) like phthalates and parabens can interfere with hormone function, potentially leading to reproductive issues, metabolic disorders, and even cancer (Gore et al., 2015). Chronic exposure to toxins can weaken the immune system, making the body more susceptible to infections and diseases (Reiche, Nunes, & Morimoto, 2004).

Detoxifying Your Home

Reducing toxin exposure in the home is crucial to creating a healthier living environment. Here are some practical tips to detoxify your home:

Using Natural Cleaning Products: Many conventional cleaning products contain toxic chemicals that can pollute indoor air and pose health risks. Switching to natural cleaning products, such as those made with vinegar, baking soda, and essential oils, can significantly reduce exposure to harmful substances (Steinemann, 2017). These natural alternatives are effective at cleaning and disinfecting without the adverse side effects associated with chemical cleaners.

Reducing Use of Plastics: Plastics, especially when heated, can release harmful chemicals like BPA and phthalates, known endocrine disruptors. To minimize exposure, reduce the use of plastic containers, especially for storing or microwaving food. Opt for glass, stainless steel, or silicone alternatives, which are safer and more sustainable (Vandenberg et al., 2007).

Improving Indoor Air Quality with Plants: Indoor air can be more polluted than outdoor air due to the accumulation of volatile organic compounds (VOCs) from household products and building materials. Houseplants like spider plants, peace lilies, and snake plants can help improve indoor air quality by absorbing toxins and releasing oxygen (Wolverton, Douglas, & Bounds, 1989). Adding these plants to your home can create a healthier environment and reduce the burden of toxins.

Detoxifying Your Diet

What we eat plays a significant role in our exposure to toxins. Making mindful choices about our diet can help reduce the intake of harmful substances.

Choosing Organic Produce: Organic produce is grown without synthetic pesticides and fertilizers, common sources of toxins in conventional farming. By choosing organic fruits and vegetables, you can reduce your exposure to these harmful chemicals (Lu et al., 2006). While organic options may be more expensive, prioritizing organic for the "Dirty Dozen" — a list of produce with the highest pesticide residues — can be cost-effective. The list identifies fruits and vegetables with the highest pesticide levels. Here are the top 12, ranked by contamination:

1 **Strawberries**
2 **Spinach**

3 Kale, collard, and mustard greens

4 Grapes

5 Peaches

6 Pears

7 Nectarines

8 Apples

9 Bell and hot peppers

10 Cherries

11 Blueberries

12 Green beans

The **Clean Fifteen** consists of fruits and vegetables with the lowest pesticide residues. When shopping for these items, you can feel more confident about conventional options:

1 Avocados

2 Sweet corn

3 Pineapples

4 Cabbages

5 Onions

6 Sweet peas (frozen)

7 Papayas

8 Asparagus

9 Mangoes

10 Eggplants

11 Honeydew melons

12 Kiwis

13 Cantaloupes

14 Cauliflower

15 Broccoli

These produce items tend to have minimal pesticide residues, making them a suitable choice even if organic versions aren't available.

Avoiding Processed Foods: Processed foods often contain artificial additives, preservatives, and unhealthy fats that can contribute to toxin buildup in the body. These substances can strain the liver and other detoxification organs, leading to long-term health issues (Monteiro et al., 2018). To detoxify your diet, focus on whole, unprocessed foods like fruits, vegetables, whole grains, and lean proteins. Preparing meals at home using fresh ingredients can also help you avoid hidden toxins.

Drinking Plenty of Water: Staying hydrated is essential for supporting the body's natural detoxification processes. Water helps flush toxins out of the body through urine, sweat, and bowel movements (Popkin, D'Anci, & Rosenberg, 2010). Aim to drink at least eight glasses of water daily, and consider using a water filter to remove contaminants like chlorine and heavy metals from your drinking water.

Detox Practices

In addition to reducing exposure to toxins in your home and diet, incorporating daily detox practices can help support your body's natural detoxification systems.

Dry Brushing for Skin Detox: Dry brushing is a practice that involves using a natural bristle brush to exfoliate the skin gently. This technique stimulates the lymphatic system, which is crucial in removing toxins from the body (McMahon, 2011). To dry brush, start at your feet and use long, sweeping motions toward your heart. This practice can help promote circulation, exfoliate dead skin cells, and support detoxification.

Epsom Salt Baths: Epsom salt baths are another effective detox practice. Epsom salts contain magnesium sulfate, which can be absorbed through the skin and help draw out toxins, reduce inflammation, and relax muscles (Kass, 2010). To prepare an Epsom salt bath, dissolve 1-2 cups of Epsom salts in warm water and soak for 20-30 minutes. This practice not only aids in detoxification but also promotes relaxation and stress relief.

Regular Physical Activity to Promote Sweating: Exercise is one of the most effective ways to support detoxification. Physical activity increases circulation, boosts the lymphatic system, and promotes sweating, which helps eliminate toxins through the skin (Scheer et al., 2010). Aim for at least 30 minutes of moderate exercise, whether walking, cycling, or yoga, most days of the week. Regular exercise can help keep your body's detoxification systems functioning optimally.

Understanding the sources of toxins and implementing strategies to reduce exposure can significantly improve your health and well-being. Detoxifying your home, diet, and daily practices helps to minimize the toxic burden on your body, allowing it to function more efficiently and supporting overall health.

4

STAYING ACTIVE AND FIT

Daily Movement Routine: Simple Exercises for Energy

Incorporating daily movement into your routine is essential for maintaining energy, promoting overall health, and enhancing your quality of life. As we age, staying active becomes even more critical for supporting bodily functions, boosting mood, and reducing the risk of chronic diseases. This section will discuss the importance of daily movement, provide a morning stretch routine to kickstart your day, suggest quick midday exercises to combat fatigue, and recommend gentle evening exercises to help you wind down.

Importance of Daily Movement

Daily movement is more than just a means of staying fit; it is a fundamental aspect of maintaining overall health and vitality. Regular physical activity offers many benefits, including improved circulation, enhanced mood, increased energy levels, and a reduced risk of chronic diseases.

Improved Circulation: Regular movement is crucial for maintaining healthy circulation. When you move, your heart pumps more efficiently, delivering oxygen and nutrients to tissues. This increased blood flow supports cellular function, promotes healing, and reduces the risk of circulatory issues such as varicose veins and blood clots (Warburton, Nicol, & Bredin, 2006). Improved circulation also helps maintain healthy skin and a youthful appearance by delivering essential nutrients to the skin cells.

Enhanced Mood: Physical activity enhances mood by stimulating the production of endorphins, the body's natural "feel-good" hormones. These endorphins help reduce feelings of stress, anxiety, and depression, contributing to a more positive outlook on life (Dunn, Trivedi, & O'Neal, 2001). Additionally, regular movement can improve self-esteem and body image, further boosting emotional well-being.

Increased Energy Levels: One of the most immediate benefits of daily movement is increased energy levels. Contrary to the common belief that physical activity can be tiring, regular exercise boosts energy by enhancing the efficiency of the cardiovascular system and improving the function of the mitochondria—the energy-producing structures in your cells (Puetz, Flowers, & O'Connor, 2008). Regular movement makes you feel more energized and capable of handling daily tasks.

Reduced Risk of Chronic Diseases: Regular physical activity is one of the most effective ways to reduce the risk of chronic diseases, including heart disease, diabetes, and osteoporosis. Exercise helps regulate blood pressure, lower cholesterol levels, and maintain healthy body weight, all contributing to a lower risk of chronic illness (Booth, Roberts, & Laye, 2012). Additionally, weight-bearing exercises help strengthen bones and reduce the risk of fractures as you age.

Morning Stretch Routine

Starting your day with a simple stretch routine can help wake up your body, improve flexibility, and set a positive tone for the day. Here's a quick morning stretch routine to kickstart your day:

Neck Stretches:

- **Instructions:** Sit or stand with your back straight. Tilt your head to the right, bringing your ear towards your shoulder. Hold for 15-20 seconds, then switch to the left side. Repeat 2-3 times on each side.

- **Benefits:** Neck stretches help relieve neck and shoulder tension, where stress commonly accumulates (Falla, Jull, & Hodges, 2004).

Shoulder Rolls:

- **Instructions:** Stand with your feet hip-width apart. Lift your shoulders towards your ears, then roll them back and down in a circular motion. Repeat ten times, then reverse the direction.

- **Benefits:** Shoulder rolls improve shoulder mobility and reduce stiffness, making them an excellent way to release tension (McQuade, Smidt, & Reid, 1998).

Gentle Spinal Twists:

- **Instructions:** Sit cross-legged on the floor or in a chair with your feet flat on the floor. Place your right hand on your left knee and twist your torso to the left, looking over your left shoulder. Hold for 15-20 seconds, then repeat on the other side.

- **Benefits:** Spinal twists help increase spinal flexibility and promote healthy digestion by massaging the abdominal organs (Wheeler & Watkins, 1988).

Hamstring Stretches:

- **Instructions:** Stand with your feet hip-width apart. Place your right foot in front of you with your heel on the ground and your toes pointing up. Hinge at your hips and reach towards your right foot, keeping your back straight. Hold for 15-20 seconds, then switch to the other leg.

- **Benefits:** Hamstring stretches improve flexibility in the back of the legs, reducing the risk of lower back pain (Worrell et al., 1991).

Midday Energy Booster

To combat midday fatigue and keep your energy levels high, incorporate quick exercises into your day. These simple movements can be done at your desk or in a small space and take just a few minutes.

Desk Stretches:

- **Instructions:** Sit up straight in your chair. Reach both arms overhead and interlace your fingers, then turn your palms towards the ceiling and stretch upwards. Hold for 10-15 seconds, then release.

Follow with a seated twist by placing one hand on the back of your chair and twisting your torso to look over your shoulder.

• **Benefits:** Desk stretches relieve tension from sitting and improve posture, helping to reduce fatigue (Thigpen et al., 2010).

Light Cardio (e.g., Marching in Place):

• **Instructions:** Stand up and march in place, lifting your knees high and swinging your arms. Continue for 1-2 minutes to raise your heart rate.

• **Benefits:** Light cardio boosts circulation and increases oxygen flow to the brain, helping to clear mental fog and improve focus (Hamer & Chida, 2008).

Breathing Exercises:

• **Instructions:** Sit comfortably and close your eyes. Inhale deeply through your nose for a count of four, hold for four, and exhale through your mouth for a count of four. Repeat for 1-2 minutes.

• **Benefits:** Deep breathing exercises increase oxygen intake, reduce stress, and refresh your mind and body (Jerath et al., 2006).

Evening Wind-Down

Gentle exercises in the evening can help you wind down and prepare your body for restful sleep. These movements promote relaxation and ease muscle tension accumulated throughout the day.

Gentle Yoga Poses (e.g., Child's Pose):

• **Instructions:** Kneel on the floor with your big toes touching and knees spread apart. Sit back on your heels and stretch your arms forward, lowering your torso towards the floor. Rest your forehead on the mat and breathe deeply for 1-2 minutes.

• **Benefits:** Child's pose is a restorative yoga pose that stretches the back, hips, and thighs while calming the mind (Browning, Lee, & Collins, 2017).

Deep Breathing Exercises:

• **Instructions:** Lie on your back with one hand on your chest and the other on your abdomen. Breathe deeply into your belly, allowing it to rise with each inhale and fall with each exhale. Continue for 5-10 minutes.

• **Benefits:** Deep breathing before bed helps activate the parasympathetic nervous system, promoting relaxation and preparing the body for sleep (Tarantino et al., 2017).

Progressive Muscle Relaxation:

• **Instructions:** Lie down in a comfortable position. Starting with your toes, tense each muscle group for 5 seconds, then release and relax. Gradually work your way up your body, from your legs to your abdomen, chest, arms, and face.

• **Benefits:** Progressive muscle relaxation helps release physical tension and reduces anxiety, aiding in a restful night's sleep (Conrad & Roth, 2007).

Incorporating these simple exercises into your daily routine can boost your energy levels, improve your mood, and support your overall health. Regular movement, whether through stretching, light cardio, or relaxation exercises, is vital in maintaining a healthy and balanced life.

Strength Training: Building Muscle and Bone Density

Strength training is essential to a well-rounded fitness routine, particularly for women over 50. Maintaining muscle mass and bone density becomes increasingly necessary as we age for overall health and quality of life. This section will explore the benefits of strength training, introduce beginner-friendly exercises, provide guidelines for creating a strength training routine, and discuss safety tips to prevent injury.

Benefits of Strength Training

Strength or resistance training involves exercises that improve muscle strength and endurance by working against resistance. This exercise particularly benefits older adults, offering various health benefits for maintaining independence and vitality.

Prevention of Muscle Loss: Muscle mass naturally declines as we age in a process known as sarcopenia. This muscle loss can lead to weakness, reduced mobility, and an increased risk of falls and fractures. Strength training helps counteract sarcopenia by stimulating muscle growth and preserving muscle mass (Hunter, McCarthy, &

Bamman, 2004). Regular strength training exercises can help maintain strength, improve physical performance, and enhance the ability to perform daily activities independently.

Improved Bone Density: Osteoporosis, a condition characterized by weakened bones and an increased risk of fractures, is a common concern for women over 50. Strength training increases bone density by stimulating the formation of new bone tissue (Layne & Nelson, 1999). Weight-bearing exercises, such as squats and resistance training, place stress on the bones, prompting them to become stronger and more resilient. Bone strength is essential for reducing the risk of fractures and maintaining bone health as we age.

Enhanced Metabolism: Strength training also plays a crucial role in boosting metabolism. Muscle tissue is metabolically active, meaning it burns more calories at rest than fat tissue (Speakman & Selman, 2003). Building and maintaining muscle mass through strength training can increase your resting metabolic rate, aiding in weight management and reducing the risk of metabolic disorders such as diabetes.

Better Balance and Coordination: Strength training improves strength and bone density and enhances balance and coordination. Exercises that target the core and lower body, such as squats and lunges, help improve stability and reduce the risk of falls (Liu-Ambrose et al., 2004). Stability is vital for older adults, as maintaining balance and coordination is essential for preventing injuries and maintaining independence.

Beginner Strength Training Exercises

For those new to strength training, it's essential to start with exercises that are accessible and safe. You can perform these beginner-friendly exercises at home or in the gym with minimal equipment:

Bodyweight Squats:

- **Instructions:** Stand with your feet shoulder-width apart, toes pointing slightly outward. Slowly bend your knees and lower your hips as if sitting back into a chair, keeping your chest up and your knees aligned with your toes. Lower yourself until your thighs are parallel to the floor, then push through your heels to return to the starting position. Repeat for 10-15 repetitions.

• **Benefits:** Squats target the muscles of the lower body, including the quadriceps, hamstrings, and glutes, and help improve balance and stability (Escamilla, 2001).

Modified Push-Ups:

• **Instructions:** Start kneeling with your hands slightly wider than shoulder-width apart on the floor. Keep your body in a straight line from your head to your knees. Lower your chest towards the floor by bending your elbows, keeping them close to your body. Push through your palms to return to the starting position. Repeat for 8-12 repetitions.

• **Benefits:** Modified push-ups strengthen the chest, shoulders, and triceps while engaging the core muscles (Cogley et al., 2005).

Resistance Band Exercises:

• **Instructions:** Use a resistance band to perform various exercises like rows and leg lifts. For rows, anchor the band at a low point and hold the handles with both hands. Stand with your feet hip-width apart and pull the handles towards your torso, squeezing your shoulder blades together. For leg lifts, loop the band around your ankles and lift one leg to the side, keeping it straight. Perform 10-15 repetitions for each exercise.

• **Benefits:** Resistance bands provide adjustable resistance and are ideal for strengthening various muscle groups while minimizing joint strain (Page, 2012).

Dumbbell Bicep Curls:

• **Instructions:** Hold a dumbbell in each hand with your arms extended by your sides, palms facing forward. Keep your elbows close to your body, bend your elbows, and curl the dumbbells towards your shoulders. Lower the dumbbells back to the starting position. Repeat for 10-15 repetitions.

• **Benefits:** Bicep curls target the biceps and help improve upper body strength, essential for everyday tasks such as lifting and carrying (Gentil, Bottaro, & Oliveira, 2017).

Creating a Strength Training Routine

When creating a strength training routine, it's essential to focus on balance, consistency, and recovery. Here are some guidelines to help you design an effective and sustainable routine:

Frequency (e.g., 2-3 times per week): For beginners, strength training 2-3 times per week is recommended, with at least one rest day between sessions to allow muscles to recover and grow (ACSM, 2009). This frequency helps build strength without overtraining, reducing the risk of injury.

Repetitions and Sets: Depending on your fitness level, start with 1-2 sets of 8-15 repetitions for each exercise. As you become stronger, you can gradually increase the number of sets or repetitions. Focus on using a weight or resistance level that allows you to complete the last repetition with good form but is challenging enough to fatigue the muscles (Kraemer et al., 2002).

Rest and Recovery: Allow 48 hours of rest between strength training sessions to give your muscles time to recover and rebuild. On rest days, incorporate light activity, such as walking or stretching, to promote circulation and reduce muscle soreness (Schoenfeld, 2010). Recovery is essential to the training process, as it helps prevent overtraining and injury.

Safety Tips

To prevent injury and ensure that you get the most out of your strength training routine, follow these safety guidelines:

Proper Warm-Up and Cool-Down: Always begin your workout with a 5-10 minute warm-up, such as brisk walking or gentle stretching, to increase blood flow to your muscles and prepare your body for exercise. After your workout, cool down with light stretching to help reduce muscle stiffness and promote flexibility (McHugh & Cosgrave, 2010).

Using Correct Form and Technique: Proper form is crucial for preventing injury and maximizing the effectiveness of each exercise. Focus on controlled movements, keep your core engaged, and avoid using momentum to lift weights. If unsure about your form, consider working with a trainer or using a mirror to check your alignment (Faigenbaum et al., 2009).

Listening to the Body and Avoiding Overexertion: Listening to your body and avoiding pushing through pain or discomfort is essential. If an exercise feels too difficult or causes pain, stop and reassess your form or try a modification. Overexertion can lead to injury, so it's essential to progress gradually and prioritize safety (Thompson et al., 2016).

By incorporating strength training into your routine, you can build and maintain muscle mass, improve bone density, enhance metabolism, and boost your overall physical health. Following these guidelines and safety tips will help you create a balanced and effective strength training program that supports your health and well-being as you age.

Cardio for Heart Health: Walking, Dancing, and More

Cardiovascular exercise, also known as cardio, is vital to a well-rounded fitness routine, particularly for maintaining heart health and overall fitness. Regular cardio activities can significantly improve cardiovascular health, increase stamina, enhance mood, and help with weight management. In this section, we will explore the importance of cardiovascular exercise, provide tips for incorporating walking into your daily routine, suggest fun dance exercises, and recommend other cardio options to keep you active and healthy.

Importance of Cardiovascular Exercise

Cardiovascular exercise is any activity that raises your heart rate and keeps it elevated for a sustained period. This exercise offers numerous essential benefits for maintaining good health, particularly as we age.

Improved Cardiovascular Health: The most significant benefit of cardiovascular exercise is its positive impact on heart health. Regular cardio strengthens the heart muscle, improves blood circulation, and helps lower blood pressure and cholesterol levels, reducing the risk of heart disease and stroke (Bassuk & Manson, 2003). Regular moderate to vigorous cardiovascular exercise is associated with lower cardiovascular events and increased longevity (Warburton, Nicol, & Bredin, 2006).

Increased Stamina and Endurance: Cardiovascular exercise also helps improve stamina and endurance by training your body to use oxygen more efficiently. Over time, this increases aerobic capacity, allowing you to perform physical activities with less fatigue and greater ease (Haskell et al., 2007). Whether climbing stairs, playing with grandchildren, or participating in recreational activities, improved endurance enhances your ability to enjoy daily life.

Enhanced Mood and Mental Health: Besides its physical benefits, cardio exercise profoundly impacts mental health. Activities like walking, dancing, and cycling release endorphins—often referred to as the body's natural "feel-good" hormones—helping to reduce stress, anxiety, and symptoms of depression (Craft & Perna, 2004). Regular cardiovascular exercise boosts mood, improves sleep quality, and enhances overall emotional well-being.

Weight Management: Cardiovascular exercise is crucial because it burns calories and boosts metabolism. Combined with a balanced diet, regular cardio can help you achieve and maintain a healthy weight, reducing the risk of obesity-related conditions such as type 2 diabetes and hypertension (Ross et al., 2000). Additionally, cardio helps reduce visceral fat, which surrounds internal organs and is linked to higher health risks.

Walking for Fitness

Walking is one of the most straightforward and accessible forms of cardiovascular exercise. It requires no special equipment, can be done almost anywhere, and is gentle on the joints, making it ideal for people of all fitness levels.

Setting a Daily Step Goal: One effective way to incorporate walking into your daily routine is by setting a step goal. Aim for 7,000 to 10,000 steps daily, roughly equivalent to 30-60 minutes of moderate-intensity walking (Tudor-Locke et al., 2011). Gradually increase your step count if you're starting from a lower baseline, and consider tracking your steps to stay motivated.

Choosing Scenic Walking Routes: To make walking more enjoyable, choose scenic routes that allow you to connect with nature or explore new areas. Parks, nature trails, and waterfront paths are attractive options that enhance the walking experience and provide additional mental health benefits through exposure to green spaces (Barton & Pretty, 2010). Mixing up your routes can also keep your routine fresh and exciting.

Using a Pedometer or Fitness Tracker: A pedometer or fitness tracker can help you monitor your progress and stay accountable to your walking goals. These devices track your steps, distance, and sometimes even your heart rate, providing valuable feedback on your activity levels (Bravata et al., 2007). Many fitness trackers also offer features like reminders to move, which can help you stay consistent with your walking routine.

Dancing for Fun and Fitness

Dancing is not only a fun way to express yourself, but it is also an effective form of cardiovascular exercise. Dancing improves heart health, builds strength, and enhances coordination while allowing you to enjoy music and socialize with others.

Zumba: Zumba is a popular dance fitness program that combines Latin and international music with energetic dance moves. It provides a full-body workout that improves cardiovascular fitness, tones muscles, and burns calories (Krishnan et al., 2015). Zumba classes are often available at gyms and community centers, or you can follow along with online videos from the comfort of your home.

Ballroom Dancing: Ballroom dancing, including styles like the waltz, foxtrot, and tango, offers a more structured form of dance exercise. It requires coordination, balance, and rhythm, making it an excellent way to improve cardiovascular health and mental sharpness (Keogh et al., 2009). Many community centers and dance studios offer classes for all skill levels, making starting easy.

Line Dancing: Line dancing involves choreographed steps performed in unison with a group, often to country or pop music. It's a fun, social activity that provides a moderate cardiovascular workout and improves balance and coordination (Noreau et al., 1995). Line dancing is viral among older adults and is often found in community centers and social clubs.

Online Dance Classes: For those who prefer to dance at home, online dance classes offer a convenient and flexible option. Platforms like YouTube or subscription-based services provide a wide variety of dance styles, from hip-hop to salsa, that you can follow at your own pace. Dancing at home allows you to customize your workout and enjoy the benefits of cardio exercise without leaving your living room.

Other Cardio Options

In addition to walking and dancing, there are many other cardio-vascular exercises that you can incorporate into your routine to keep things varied and engaging.

Swimming: Swimming is a low-impact cardio exercise that is gentle on the joints while providing a full-body workout. It improves cardiovascular fitness, builds endurance, and strengthens muscles, making it an excellent option for people with arthritis or other joint issues (Lee & Oh, 2013). Swimming laps, participating in water aerobics, or simply treading water can improve heart health.

Cycling: Cycling is another effective form of cardio exercise, whether on a stationary bike or outdoors. It strengthens the legs, improves cardiovascular endurance, and can be enjoyed at different fitness levels (Oja et al., 2011). Cycling outdoors also allows you to explore new areas and enjoy the scenery, adding an element of adventure to your workout.

Hiking: Hiking combines the benefits of walking with the added challenge of varying terrain, making it a great way to build cardiovascular fitness and strengthen the lower body (Ettema & Lorås, 2012). Hiking in nature also offers mental health benefits, such as reducing stress and improving mood. Whether you choose a gentle trail or a more challenging hike, this activity provides an excellent workout.

Low-Impact Aerobics: Low-impact aerobics classes provide a cardiovascular workout without the high-impact movements that can strain the joints. These classes often include exercises like marching, step touches, and gentle lunges, set to music to keep the workout enjoyable (Schlicht et al., 2001). Low-impact aerobics is ideal for older adults or those new to exercise, as it improves fitness while minimizing the risk of injury.

By incorporating various cardiovascular exercises into your routine, such as walking, dancing, swimming, and cycling, you can improve your heart health, boost your mood, and enhance your overall fitness. These activities are not only beneficial for your physical health but also offer enjoyable ways to stay active and engaged.

Flexibility and Balance: Preventing Falls and Injuries

Maintaining flexibility and balance is essential for preventing falls and injuries, especially as we age. These two components of physical fitness contribute to enhanced mobility, improved posture, and greater ease in performing daily activities. This section will discuss the benefits of flexibility and balance, provide instructions for critical exercises, and offer tips for integrating these practices into your daily routine.

Benefits of Flexibility and Balance

Maintaining flexibility and balance becomes increasingly important for overall health and safety as we age. These aspects of fitness enhance mobility and play a critical role in preventing falls and injuries, which can have severe consequences for older adults.

Enhanced Mobility: Flexibility allows for a greater range of motion in the joints, which is crucial for performing everyday activities efficiently, such as reaching, bending, and walking (Hunter, Whitehead, & McGregor, 2008). Regular stretching helps maintain or improve joint flexibility, making moving easier without discomfort or stiffness. Enhanced mobility also supports physical independence, allowing you to enjoy various activities as you age.

Reduced Risk of Falls: Falls are a leading cause of injury among older adults, often resulting in fractures, hospitalizations, and a decline in quality of life (Ambrose, Paul, & Hausdorff, 2013). Maintaining good balance is critical to preventing falls, as it helps you stay steady on your feet and recover quickly from any slips or stumbles.

Incorporating balance exercises into your routine strengthens the muscles that stabilize your body, reducing the likelihood of falls.

Improved Posture: Good posture is essential for overall health and well-being. It helps align the body properly, reducing strain on muscles and joints and preventing discomfort or injury. Flexibility exercises, particularly those that target the spine, shoulders, and hips, can help correct postural imbalances and promote a more upright and confident stance (Kendall, McCreary, & Provance, 2005). Improved posture also contributes to better breathing, digestion, and circulation.

Greater Ease in Daily Activities: Maintaining flexibility and balance can make daily activities more manageable and enjoyable. Whether it's bending down to pick something up, reaching for an item on a high shelf, or simply walking up stairs, these exercises ensure that your body is prepared to handle the physical demands of everyday life (Shumway-Cook & Woollacott, 2007). This ease of movement enhances your independence and helps you maintain a high quality of life.

Flexibility Exercises

Incorporating flexibility exercises into your routine is essential for maintaining joint mobility and preventing stiffness. Here are some critical exercises to improve flexibility:

Hamstring Stretches:

• **Instructions:** Sit on the floor with your legs extended straight in front of you. Slowly reach forward with both hands towards your toes, keeping your back straight. Hold the stretch for 20-30 seconds, then relax. Repeat 2-3 times.

• **Benefits:** Hamstring stretches improve flexibility in the back of the legs, reducing the risk of lower back pain and enhancing mobility in activities like walking and bending (Worrell et al., 1991).

Hip Flexor Stretches:

• **Instructions:** Kneel on one knee with the other foot in front, forming a 90-degree angle at both knees. Gently push your hips forward while keeping your back straight, feeling a stretch in the front of the hip. Hold for 20-30 seconds, then switch sides. Repeat 2-3 times.

• **Benefits:** Hip flexor stretches help relieve tightness in the hips, improving posture and reducing strain on the lower back (Neelly, Noble, & Etnyre, 1992).

Shoulder Stretches:

• **Instructions:** Extend one arm across your body at shoulder height. Use your opposite hand to gently pull the extended arm closer to your chest. Hold for 20-30 seconds, then switch sides. Repeat 2-3 times.

• **Benefits:** Shoulder stretches increase flexibility in the shoulder joints and upper back, helping to improve posture and reduce the risk of shoulder injuries (McClure et al., 2007).

Seated Forward Bends:

• **Instructions:** Sit on the floor with your legs extended in front of you. Slowly hinge at your hips and reach towards your toes, keeping your back straight. Hold the stretch for 20-30 seconds, then relax. Repeat 2-3 times.

• **Benefits:** Seated forward bends stretch the lower back, hamstrings, and calves, promoting flexibility in the spine and legs (Boone & Azen, 1979).

Balance Exercises

Balance exercises are crucial for improving stability and reducing the risk of falls. Here are some exercises specifically designed to enhance balance:

Standing on One Leg:

• **Instructions:** Stand near a wall or sturdy chair for support. Lift one foot off the ground and balance on the other leg. Hold the position for 20-30 seconds, then switch legs. Repeat 2-3 times on each leg. To increase difficulty, try closing your eyes or moving your arms.

• **Benefits:** Standing on one leg strengthens the lower body and core muscles, improving stability and balance (Orr et al., 2008).

Heel-to-Toe Walk:

• **Instructions:** Walk in a straight line by placing the heel of one foot directly in front of the toes of the other foot. Continue walking in this manner for 10-15 steps. For added support, use a wall or railing for balance.

• **Benefits:** The heel-to-toe walk improves balance and coordination by challenging your stability as you move (Shumway-Cook & Woollacott, 2007).

Balance Exercises Using a Stability Ball:

• **Instructions:** Sit on a stability ball with your feet flat on the floor, hip-width apart. Engage your core and lift one foot off the ground, holding the position for 10-15 seconds. Switch legs and repeat. For an added challenge, try lifting both feet off the ground simultaneously.

• **Benefits:** Using a stability ball improves core strength and balance by requiring constant adjustments to maintain stability (Behm et al., 2005).

Tai Chi Movements:

• **Instructions:** Practice simple Tai Chi movements such as "Wave Hands Like Clouds" or "Golden Rooster Stands on One Leg." These slow, controlled movements emphasize weight shifting and balance. Join a Tai Chi class or follow along with an instructional video.

• **Benefits:** Tai Chi enhances balance, coordination, and flexibility and reduces the risk of falls in older adults (Gatts & Woollacott, 2006).

Incorporating Flexibility and Balance into Daily Life

Incorporating flexibility and balance exercises into your daily routine doesn't have to be time-consuming. Here are some tips for integrating these practices into everyday activities:

Stretching During TV Commercials: Use commercial breaks to perform quick stretches. For example, stand up and do a hamstring or shoulder stretch while watching your favorite show. Fit stretching into your day without setting aside dedicated time (Griffin et al., 2014).

Balance Exercises While Brushing Teeth: Practice standing on one leg or performing heel-to-toe walks while brushing your teeth. This simple habit can help improve your balance without requiring extra time or effort (Stevens et al., 2012).

Gentle Stretches Before Bed: Incorporate a few minutes of gentle stretching into your bedtime routine. Stretching before bed can help relax muscles, reduce tension, and promote better sleep (Mejía-Mejía et al., 2020).

Incorporating flexibility and balance exercises into your daily routine regularly can enhance your mobility, reduce the risk of falls, and improve your overall quality of life. These practices are essential for maintaining independence and staying active as you age.

Fun and Fitness: Enjoyable Activities to Stay Active

Staying active is crucial for maintaining physical health and provides joy and social connection. Choosing enjoyable activities is critical to sustaining a long-term fitness routine, as it transforms exercise from a chore into a fun and rewarding part of daily life. This section will explore the importance of combining fun with fitness, suggest group activities that promote social interaction, recommend outdoor adventures for physical fitness, and provide creative home exercise ideas.

Combining Fun and Fitness

One of the most effective ways to ensure consistency in your fitness routine is to choose activities you genuinely enjoy. When exercise is fun, staying motivated and committed is easier, leading to many physical and mental health benefits.

Increased Adherence to Fitness Routines: Enjoyable activities are more likely to become regular habits. Research shows that people who enjoy their exercise routines are likelier to stick with them over the long term (Kinnafick, Thøgersen-Ntoumani, & Duda, 2014). This increased adherence is crucial for reaping the full benefits of physical activity, including improved cardiovascular health, enhanced muscle tone, and better overall fitness.

Reduced Perception of Exercise as a Chore: When fitness activities are enjoyable, they no longer feel like a mandatory task or chore. Instead, they become something to look forward to, reducing the mental barrier often accompanying traditional exercise routines

(Ryan et al., 1997). This shift in perception can make incorporating physical activity into your daily life easier.

Enhanced Mental Well-Being: Engaging in fun physical activities can boost mood and reduce stress. The enjoyment derived from these activities releases endorphins, which are natural mood elevators (Craft & Perna, 2004). Moreover, fun fitness activities can serve as mindfulness, helping to clear the mind and focus on the present moment, further enhancing mental well-being.

Opportunities for Social Interaction: Choosing group activities or social sports can provide valuable opportunities for social interaction. This social aspect makes exercise more enjoyable and contributes to emotional health by fostering a sense of community and belonging (Bailey, 2005). Regular social interaction has been linked to lower rates of depression and anxiety, making it an essential component of overall health.

Group Activities

Group fitness activities offer the dual benefits of physical exercise and social interaction. Here are some group activities that promote both enjoyment and fitness:

Group Hiking Trips: Hiking with a group allows one to enjoy nature, engage in moderate to vigorous physical activity, and socialize. Group hikes can be organized through local hiking clubs, community centers, or informal gatherings of friends. Hiking strengthens the legs and cardiovascular system and promotes mental relaxation through exposure to natural environments (Mitchell, Bennett, & Manfred, 2013).

Water Aerobics Classes: Water aerobics is a low-impact exercise particularly beneficial for older adults and those with joint issues. Participating in a water aerobics class provides a full-body workout while minimizing joint stress (Colado et al., 2009). The group setting also fosters camaraderie and motivation, making it enjoyable to stay active.

Group Cycling: Cycling with a group is an excellent way to combine cardiovascular exercise with social interaction. Many communities have cycling clubs or groups that organize regular rides for various skill levels. Group cycling improves fitness, encourages safe riding practices, and provides a support network for participants (Oja et al., 2011).

Community Fitness Challenges: Participating in community fitness challenges, such as charity walks, fun runs, or local sports tournaments, can be a motivating way to stay active while contributing to a more significant cause. These events often have a festive atmosphere, making exercise feel like a celebration rather than a task. The sense of achievement from completing a challenge can also boost self-esteem and encourage continued participation in fitness activities (Baker, 2010).

Outdoor Adventures

Engaging in outdoor activities is a fantastic way to stay active while enjoying the beauty of nature. These activities are physically beneficial and provide mental and emotional rewards.

Kayaking: Kayaking offers a full-body workout that strengthens the arms, shoulders, back, and core while providing a peaceful and scenic experience on the water. Whether paddling on a lake, river, or ocean, kayaking can be a meditative activity that allows you to connect with nature while staying physically active (Caldwell et al., 2012).

Gardening: Gardening is a surprisingly effective form of physical exercise that involves bending, lifting, digging, and stretching. It's a low-impact activity that can improve strength, flexibility, and endurance. Additionally, gardening offers the mental health benefits of spending time outdoors and nurturing living plants, which can reduce stress and increase feelings of well-being (Relf, 1992).

Birdwatching Walks: Birdwatching walks combine the benefits of gentle walking with the mindfulness of observing wildlife. These walks can be done alone or with a group and provide a way to stay active while enjoying the sights and sounds of nature. Birdwatching also encourages focus and patience, making it a mentally engaging activity (Cooper & Smith, 2019).

Geocaching: Geocaching is a modern-day treasure hunt that involves using GPS to find hidden containers, or "geocaches," in outdoor locations. It's a fun and adventurous way to explore new areas, walk or hike, and engage in problem-solving. Geocaching can be enjoyed alone, with friends, or as a family activity, making it a versatile option for staying active (O'Hara, 2008).

Creative Home Exercises

Staying active at home doesn't have to be monotonous. You can turn your home into a fun and dynamic fitness environment with some creativity.

Dance Parties with Favorite Music: Turn up the volume on your favorite songs and have a dance party in your living room. Dancing is a great cardiovascular workout that improves coordination, balance, and mood. Plus, dancing to music you love can make exercise feel like a celebration rather than a routine (Moe, 2014).

Virtual Fitness Challenges with Friends: Challenge your friends to virtual fitness competitions, such as who can take the most steps in a week or complete the most workout sessions. These challenges can be tracked using fitness apps, adding a competitive and social element to your exercise routine. The accountability and camaraderie of virtual challenges can help keep you motivated (Maher et al., 2016).

Exercise Games with Grandchildren: If you have grandchildren, involve them in your fitness routine by playing active games together. Games like tag, hide-and-seek, or a simple obstacle course can give you and your grandchildren physical exercise while fostering bonding time. These activities are fun and help instill the value of physical fitness in younger generations (Pate et al., 1997).

You can make fitness a fun and integral part of your life by choosing activities you enjoy, whether in a group setting, outdoors, or at home. These enjoyable activities promote physical health, mental well-being, and social connection, ensuring you stay active and engaged at any age.

Creating a Home Gym: Essential Equipment and Tips

Creating a home gym offers numerous advantages for those seeking a convenient and consistent fitness routine. A well-equipped home gym provides the flexibility to exercise on your schedule, in a personalized environment, and without the recurring costs of gym memberships. In this section, we will explore the benefits of a home gym, suggest essential equipment for a versatile workout space, provide tips for setting up your gym, and discuss critical safety considerations.

Benefits of a Home Gym

A home gym offers several key advantages, making it an attractive option for maintaining a regular fitness routine.

No Need for Gym Membership: One of the most significant benefits of a home gym is eliminating the need for a gym membership. Over time, gym memberships can become costly, especially if you're paying for features or classes you don't use regularly. By investing in a home gym, you make a one-time purchase that can serve you for years, saving money in the long run (Graves & Kroll, 2000).

Flexibility in Workout Schedule: A home gym provides the ultimate flexibility in your workout schedule. You can exercise whenever it suits you—early in the morning, late at night, or even during a lunch break—without being constrained by the operating hours of a traditional gym. This flexibility is particularly beneficial for those with busy schedules or irregular working hours (Bailey, 2015).

Personalized Workout Environment: With a home gym, you have complete control over your workout environment. You can choose the equipment, music, and ambiance that best motivate you, creating a space uniquely tailored to your preferences. This personalized environment can make exercise more enjoyable and reduce the likelihood of skipping workouts (Haskell et al., 2007).

Cost-Effective in the Long Run: While the initial investment in home gym equipment might seem significant, it can be more cost-effective over time. A home gym can save money in the long run by eliminating monthly gym fees and reducing travel time and costs. Additionally, the equipment you purchase will typically last for many years, providing ongoing value (Laukkanen et al., 2007).

Essential Home Gym Equipment

When setting up a home gym, choosing versatile equipment that allows you to perform a wide range of exercises is important. Here's a list of essential items that can help you create a comprehensive workout space:

Resistance Bands:

• **Description:** Resistance bands are lightweight, portable, and versatile equipment that can be used for strength training, stretching, and rehabilitation exercises. They come in various resistance levels, making them suitable for all fitness levels (Page, 2012).

• **Benefits:** Resistance bands are an excellent alternative to weights and can target every major muscle group. They're also great for adding variety to your workouts and can easily be stored away when not in use.

Dumbbells:

• **Description:** Dumbbells are a staple in any home gym, offering a wide range of strength training options. They come in various weights, allowing for progressive resistance as you build strength (Kraemer & Ratamess, 2004).

• **Benefits:** Dumbbells are ideal for bicep curls, tricep extensions, shoulder presses, and chest flies. They help improve muscle tone and increase strength and are versatile enough to be used in numerous exercises.

Yoga Mat:

• **Description:** A yoga mat provides a comfortable and non-slip surface for floor exercises, yoga, and stretching routines. It's essential for activities that require stability and cushioning, such as Pilates or bodyweight exercises (Jenkins et al., 2015).

• **Benefits:** A good quality yoga mat protects your joints during exercises and provides a clean, cushioned area for floor-based activities. It's also easy to roll up and store when not in use.

Stability Ball:

- **Description:** A stability ball, also known as a Swiss ball, is a large, inflatable ball used for strength training, balance exercises, and core stabilization. It's particularly effective for engaging the abdominal muscles and improving overall balance (Behm et al., 2005).
- **Benefits:** Stability balls are versatile tools for exercises like ball squats, planks, and stability ball crunches. They add an element of instability to your workouts, making your muscles work harder to maintain balance.

Jump Rope:

- **Description:** A jump rope is a simple yet highly effective piece of cardio equipment. It provides a full-body workout and improves cardiovascular fitness, coordination, and agility (Schenk et al., 2016).
- **Benefits:** Jumping rope is a quick way to elevate your heart rate and burn calories. It's an excellent warm-up tool or can be used for high-intensity interval training (HIIT) sessions.

Setting Up Your Space

Creating a practical and motivating home gym space involves more than just purchasing equipment. Here are some tips for setting up your home gym:

Choosing a Dedicated Workout Area: Select a specific area in your home to dedicate to your workouts. This could be a spare room, a section of the garage, or even a corner of your living room. A dedicated space helps mentally prepare you for exercise and keeps your equipment organized and easily accessible (Bailey, 2015).

Ensuring Proper Lighting and Ventilation: Good lighting is essential for creating an inviting workout environment and ensuring you can safely perform exercises. Natural light is ideal, but invest in bright, energy-efficient lighting if that's impossible. Proper ventilation is also crucial for maintaining air quality and keeping the space comfortable during workouts. Consider adding a fan or air purifier if needed (Haskell et al., 2007).

Adding Motivational Elements (e.g., Posters, Music): Enhance your workout space with motivational elements like fitness posters, mirrors, or a sound system for playing your favorite music. These elements boost your energy, keep you focused, and make your workouts more enjoyable. Surrounding yourself with positive visuals and sounds can help you stay committed to your fitness goals (Ryan et al., 1997).

Home Gym Safety

Working out at home requires careful attention to safety to prevent injuries and ensure that your exercises are practical.

Keeping the Workout Area Clutter-Free: A clutter-free workout space is essential for safety. Ensure your exercise area is clear of obstacles, cords, and loose equipment that could cause tripping or accidents. Clear space is necessary when performing exercises involving quick movements or direction changes (Oja et al., 2011).

Properly Storing Equipment: After each workout, take the time to store your equipment correctly. Resistance bands, dumbbells, and other gear should be put away in designated areas to prevent damage and keep the space organized. Using storage racks, shelves, or bins can help keep your home gym tidy and reduce the risk of accidents (Page, 2012).

Monitoring Form and Technique: When working out at home, you must be mindful of your form and technique to avoid injury. Use mirrors or record yourself to check your posture and alignment during exercises. If you're unsure about proper form, consider using online tutorials or virtual sessions with a personal trainer to ensure you perform exercises correctly (Schenk et al., 2016).

By creating a home gym with essential equipment, setting up a motivating space, and following safety guidelines, you can enjoy the convenience and flexibility of working out at home. This personalized workout environment will help you stay consistent with your fitness routine, providing long-term health benefits.

PLEASE SHARE

If you have found value in this book, please share your experience by leaving a rating or a review on Amazon.

If you are reading an ebook, please click this link to be taken to your review page.

If you are reading a print book, point your phone's camera at the QR code below to be taken to your review page.

Thank you!

5

MENTAL AND EMOTIONAL WELL-BEING

Brain-Boosting Activities: Keeping Your Mind Sharp

Maintaining cognitive health becomes increasingly important as we age for overall well-being and quality of life. Engaging in brain-boosting activities is essential to keeping the mind sharp, enhancing memory and attention, and reducing the risk of cognitive decline. This section will explore the importance of cognitive health, suggest various puzzles and games that stimulate the brain, encourage learning new skills, and recommend specific brain training apps.

Importance of Cognitive Health

Cognitive health refers to thinking clearly, learning new information, and remembering important details. Like any other organ, the brain changes as we age, affecting these cognitive functions. However, regular mental exercises can help maintain cognitive health and reduce the risk of decline.

Reduced Risk of Cognitive Decline: One of the most compelling reasons to focus on cognitive health is to reduce the risk of cognitive decline, including conditions like dementia and Alzheimer's disease.

Studies have shown that engaging in mentally stimulating activities can help protect the brain from the effects of aging and slow the progression of cognitive impairment (Wilson et al., 2002). Keeping the brain active through various forms of mental exercise helps build cognitive reserve, which can delay the onset of cognitive decline (Stern, 2009).

Enhanced Memory and Attention: Regular cognitive activities protect against decline and enhance memory and attention. Activities that challenge the brain, such as puzzles and learning new skills, improve neural connections and increase brain plasticity, leading to better memory retention and sharper attention spans (Park & Bischof, 2013). Mental gymnastics can improve daily functioning, learning, and retaining new information.

Improved Problem-Solving Skills: Cognitive problem-solving exercises can significantly enhance critical thinking and decision-making abilities. Engaging in activities that require strategic thinking or solving complex problems helps keep the brain agile and improves its ability to process information quickly and accurately (Basak et al., 2008). These skills are crucial for navigating the challenges of everyday life and maintaining independence as we age.

Engaging in Puzzles and Games

Puzzles and games are enjoyable ways to keep the brain active and engaged. They offer mental challenges that stimulate different brain areas, helping to improve memory, attention, and problem-solving skills.

Crossword Puzzles: Crossword puzzles are a classic brain exercise that challenges vocabulary, memory, and problem-solving skills. Regularly completing crossword puzzles has been associated with improved cognitive function and a reduced risk of memory loss (Verghese et al., 2003). They require you to recall words and phrases, making them an excellent workout for the brain.

Sudoku: Sudoku puzzles are another excellent way to keep the brain sharp. This number-based puzzle requires logical thinking and pattern recognition, which helps improve concentration and cognitive flexibility (Gobet & Clarkson, 2004). Sudoku can be easily incorporated into your daily routine, whether in the morning with coffee or before bed.

Jigsaw Puzzles: Jigsaw puzzles are beneficial for enhancing visual-spatial reasoning and memory. Completing a jigsaw puzzle requires you to recognize patterns, piece together parts of a whole, and think critically about where each piece fits. This type of puzzle helps strengthen connections between brain cells, improving mental speed and thought processes (Lewis et al., 2015).

Strategy Board Games (e.g., Chess): Strategy board games like chess require strategic thinking, planning, and foresight, making them excellent tools for cognitive enhancement. Playing chess has been shown to improve memory, problem-solving skills, and cognitive function in older adults (Sala et al., 2017). These games engage multiple brain areas, making them highly effective for maintaining mental sharpness.

Learning New Skills

Learning new skills is one of the most effective ways to stimulate brain function and strengthen cognitive abilities. It challenges the brain to adapt, learn, and grow, which is essential for cognitive health.

Learning a New Language: Learning a new language is a highly effective way to boost cognitive health. It engages multiple brain areas, including memory, attention, and problem-solving. Research has shown that bilingualism can delay the onset of dementia and enhance cognitive reserve (Bialystok, Craik, & Luk, 2012). Language learning apps, classes, or even practicing with a language partner can be beneficial.

Taking Up a Musical Instrument: Playing a musical instrument is another powerful way to stimulate the brain. It requires coordination, memory, and concentration, strengthening neural pathways. Studies have shown that playing an instrument can improve cognitive function, enhance memory, and even increase IQ (Schellenberg, 2004). Learning to play music, whether the piano, guitar or another instrument, can be rewarding and mentally stimulating.

Enrolling in Online Courses: Enrolling in online courses allows you to continue learning and challenging your brain well into advanced adulthood. Many platforms offer classes on various subjects, from history and science to art and technology. Lifelong learning through formal education improves cognitive function and lowers the risk of cognitive decline (Elias et al., 2000). Online courses provide the flexibility to learn at your own pace and on topics that interest you.

Brain Training Apps

In addition to traditional methods of cognitive exercise, brain training apps offer a modern approach to keeping the mind sharp. These apps improve specific cognitive skills, such as memory, attention, and problem-solving, through interactive games and exercises.

Lumosity: Lumosity is a popular brain training app with various games designed to improve cognitive abilities. The app tailors its exercises to your strengths and weaknesses, providing a personalized training program that can help enhance memory, attention, and flexibility (Hardy et al., 2015).

Elevate: Elevate focuses on skills related to reading, writing, and math, offering games that challenge cognitive abilities in these areas. The app is designed to improve communication skills, processing speed, and problem-solving abilities, making it a comprehensive tool for cognitive enhancement (Mackey et al., 2012).

Peak: Peak offers a variety of fun and challenging brain training games. The app tracks your progress over time, allowing you to see improvements in areas such as memory, attention, and problem-solving. Peak is particularly effective for those looking to maintain or improve cognitive health as they age (Owen et al., 2010).

By incorporating these brain-boosting activities into your daily routine, you can maintain cognitive health, improve memory and problem-solving skills, and reduce the risk of cognitive decline. Whether through puzzles, learning new skills, or using brain training apps, there are many ways to keep your mind sharp and engaged as you age.

Managing Stress: Techniques for a Calm Mind

Stress is an inevitable part of life, but chronic stress can have significant adverse effects on both the body and mind. Understanding how stress affects you and learning effective management techniques can improve your overall well-being. This section will explain the nature of stress, provide instructions for practical breathing exercises, suggest mindfulness and meditation practices, and recommend various tools and resources for managing stress.

Understanding Stress

Stress is the body's response to any demand or challenge that disrupts its normal balance. While stress can sometimes be beneficial by providing the energy and focus needed to handle difficult situations, chronic stress can severely affect physical and emotional health.

Physical Symptoms: When the body is under stress, it triggers the "fight or flight" response, releasing hormones like adrenaline and cortisol. While this response is helpful in short bursts, prolonged activation can lead to physical symptoms such as headaches, fatigue, muscle tension, and digestive issues (McEwen, 2006). Chronic stress has also can cause more severe conditions such as cardiovascular disease, hypertension, and weakened immune function (Cohen et al., 2007).

Emotional Symptoms: Stress doesn't just affect the body; it also takes a toll on emotional health. Common emotional symptoms of stress include anxiety, irritability, mood swings, and difficulty concentrating. Over time, unmanaged stress can contribute to mental health issues like depression and anxiety disorders (Kendler et al., 2010). Recognizing and addressing these symptoms early through effective stress management techniques is crucial for maintaining emotional well-being.

Long-Term Health Impacts: The long-term impacts of chronic stress are profound, affecting nearly every system in the body. Prolonged exposure to stress can lead to burnout, characterized by physical and emotional exhaustion, detachment, and ineffectiveness. Chronic stress has also been linked to the development of chronic illnesses such as diabetes, obesity, and autoimmune diseases (Schneiderman, Ironson, & Siegel, 2005). Managing stress effectively is therefore essential for mental health and preventing long-term physical health problems.

Breathing Techniques

Breathing exercises are a simple yet powerful tool for managing stress. They help calm the nervous system, reduce anxiety, and promote relaxation. Here are some effective breathing techniques to incorporate into your stress management routine:

Deep Belly Breathing:

• **Instructions:** Sit or lie down in a comfortable position. Place one hand on your chest and the other on your abdomen. Inhale deeply through your nose, allowing your abdomen to rise as you fill your lungs with air. Exhale slowly through your mouth, letting your abdomen fall. Focus on breathing deeply and thoroughly rather than shallowly from your chest. Repeat for 5-10 minutes.

• **Benefits:** Deep belly breathing, also known as diaphragmatic breathing, helps lower cortisol levels and activate the body's relaxation response, making it an effective technique for reducing stress and anxiety (Conrad, Müller, Doberenz, & et al., 2007).

4-7-8 Breathing Technique:

• **Instructions:** Begin by inhaling quietly through your nose for a count of four. Hold your breath for a count of seven. Then, exhale completely through your mouth, making a whooshing sound for a count of eight. Repeat this cycle four times.

• **Benefits:** The 4-7-8 breathing technique helps reduce stress by slowing the heart rate and promoting relaxation. It's beneficial for calming the mind before sleep (Weil, 2011).

Alternate Nostril Breathing:

• **Instructions:** Sit comfortably and place your left hand on your left knee. Use your right thumb to close your right nostril. Inhale deeply through your left nostril, then close it with your right ring finger. Open your right nostril and exhale through it. Inhale through the right nostril, close it with your right thumb, then exhale through the left nostril. Continue alternating for 5-10 minutes.

- **Benefits:** Alternate nostril breathing, a practice rooted in yoga, balances the right and left hemispheres of the brain, reduces stress, and enhances focus and mental clarity (Telles, Singh, & Balkrishna, 2011).

Mindfulness and Meditation

Mindfulness and meditation practices are highly effective for managing stress and promoting mental well-being. These practices help you stay grounded in the present moment, reducing anxiety and improving emotional regulation.

Guided Meditations: Guided meditations involve following a narrator or instructor through a structured meditation practice. These meditations can focus on various themes, such as relaxation, self-compassion, or stress reduction. Many guided meditations are available through apps like Calm or Headspace or on platforms like YouTube (Goyal et al., 2014). Regular practice can help reduce stress, improve focus, and enhance overall emotional health.

Mindful Walking: Mindful walking is a form of meditation that involves paying close attention to the sensations of walking, such as the feeling of your feet touching the ground, the rhythm of your breath, and the sights and sounds around you. You can do this in a park, on a quiet street, or indoors. Mindful walking helps reduce stress by shifting your focus away from worries and onto the present moment (Sharma & Rush, 2014).

Body Scan Meditation: Body scan meditation is a mindfulness practice that involves mentally scanning your body from head to toe, paying attention to any sensations, tension, or areas of discomfort. Start by focusing on your toes, then gradually move up through your legs, torso, arms, and head. This practice helps release physical tension, calm the mind, and promote relaxation (Kabat-Zinn, 1990). It's handy for reducing stress and improving sleep quality.

Stress Management Tools

In addition to breathing exercises and mindfulness practices, various tools and resources are available to help manage stress effectively.

Stress Relief Journals: Keeping a stress relief journal can be an effective way to manage stress. Writing down your thoughts, feelings, and experiences helps to process emotions and gain perspective on stressful situations. You can also use journaling to track stressors and identify patterns, making it easier to develop strategies for managing stress (Pennebaker & Chung, 2011).

Stress Management Apps: Several apps can help manage stress by providing guided meditations, breathing exercises, and other relaxation techniques. Apps like Calm and Headspace offer a variety of tools for reducing stress, improving sleep, and enhancing mindfulness (Bostock, Crosswell, Prather, & Steptoe, 2019). These apps are convenient and accessible, making incorporating stress management practices into your daily routine effortless.

Aromatherapy Diffusers: Aromatherapy uses essential oils to promote relaxation and reduce stress. An aromatherapy diffuser can disperse calming scents like lavender, chamomile, or eucalyptus throughout your home. Inhaling these scents can help reduce anxiety, improve mood, and promote a sense of calm (Cavanagh & Wilkinson, 2002). Aromatherapy can be used with other stress management techniques in a holistic approach to well-being.

By understanding stress and using these techniques and tools, you can effectively manage stress and maintain a calm mind. Regularly practicing these stress management strategies will help you navigate life's challenges with greater resilience and peace of mind.

Emotional Resilience: Handling the Ups and Downs of Life

Emotional resilience is adapting to and recovering from life's challenges and adversities. It is crucial for maintaining mental and emotional well-being, particularly as we navigate life's inevitable ups and downs. This section will explore the importance of emotional resilience, provide practical coping strategies, discuss the role of gratitude in enhancing resilience, and recommend therapeutic techniques to build emotional strength.

Building Emotional Resilience

Emotional resilience is coping with stress, adversity, and change while maintaining psychological well-being. It enables individuals to bounce back from difficult situations and continue moving forward.

Ability to Bounce Back from Adversity: One critical aspect of emotional resilience is the ability to recover quickly from setbacks and challenges. Resilient individuals are not immune to stress or hardship; they have developed the tools to manage and overcome these difficulties. Research shows that emotionally resilient people can better maintain a positive outlook and recover from traumatic events or significant life changes (Bonanno, 2004). This ability to bounce back is essential for long-term mental health and well-being.

Enhanced Emotional Regulation: Emotional resilience also involves regulating one's emotions in the face of stress and being able to manage feelings of anger, sadness, or frustration without becoming overwhelmed. Resilient individuals are more likely to use adaptive coping strategies, such as reframing negative thoughts or practicing relaxation techniques, which help them maintain emotional balance (Tugade & Fredrickson, 2004). Enhanced emotional regulation improves decision-making, relationships, and overall mental health.

Greater Life Satisfaction: Resilience leads to greater life satisfaction. Emotionally resilient people experience higher happiness and contentment because they are better equipped to handle life's inevitable challenges. They are more likely to view obstacles as opportunities for growth rather than insurmountable barriers (Luthar, Cicchetti, & Becker, 2000). This positive mindset fosters a sense of purpose and fulfillment, leading to a more satisfying and meaningful life.

Coping Strategies

Developing effective coping strategies is essential for building and maintaining emotional resilience. These strategies help individuals manage stress, navigate challenges, and support emotional well-being.

Practicing Self-Compassion: Self-compassion involves treating oneself with kindness and understanding rather than being overly critical or judgmental during times of difficulty. It is a powerful coping strategy that fosters resilience by promoting self-acceptance and reducing feelings of shame or inadequacy (Neff, 2003). Self-compassionate individuals are more likely to acknowledge their struggles without feeling defeated, which enables them to recover more quickly from setbacks.

Developing a Growth Mindset: A growth mindset is the belief that the individual can develop intelligence and abilities through effort and learning. This mindset encourages individuals to view challenges as opportunities for growth rather than threats to their self-worth (Dweck, 2006). Adopting a growth mindset makes people more likely to persist in adversity, learn from their experiences, and ultimately become more resilient.

Seeking Social Support: Social support is a critical component of emotional resilience. A network of supportive friends, family members, or community resources can provide comfort, advice, and encouragement during difficult times. Research shows that individuals with strong social connections are better able to cope with stress and are less likely to experience adverse mental health outcomes (Cohen & Wills, 1985). Building and maintaining these relationships is essential for long-term resilience.

Gratitude Practices

Practicing gratitude is a powerful way to enhance emotional resilience. Individuals can cultivate a more optimistic and resilient mindset by focusing on the positive aspects of life, even during challenging times.

Keeping a Gratitude Journal: One effective way to practice gratitude is to keep a gratitude journal and regularly write down things for which you are thankful, big or small. Gratitude journaling improves mood, increases life satisfaction, and enhances emotional resilience by shifting focus away from negative experiences and towards positive ones (Emmons & McCullough, 2003). Regularly reflecting on the good things in life can help build a more resilient mindset.

Daily Gratitude Reflections: Besides journaling, taking a few moments each day to reflect on what you are grateful for can also strengthen resilience. Giving thanks in the morning sets a positive tone for the day. By making gratitude a daily habit, individuals can train their minds to focus on positivity, even in adversity (Wood, Froh, & Geraghty, 2010).

Sharing Gratitude with Others: Expressing gratitude to others, whether through verbal acknowledgment, written notes, or acts of kindness, can also enhance emotional resilience. Sharing gratitude strengthens relationships and reinforces positive emotions, creating a cycle of positivity and support (Algoe, Haidt, & Gable, 2008). This social aspect of gratitude can further bolster resilience by fostering more robust connections with others.

Therapeutic Techniques

In addition to personal practices, specific therapeutic techniques can help build emotional resilience. These approaches provide structured ways to develop coping skills, enhance emotional regulation, and foster a resilient mindset.

Cognitive-Behavioral Therapy (CBT) Exercises: Cognitive-behavioral therapy (CBT) is a widely used therapeutic approach that focuses on identifying and challenging negative thought patterns and behaviors. CBT exercises help individuals reframe negative thoughts, develop healthier coping mechanisms, and improve emotional regulation (Beck, 2011). By practicing CBT techniques, individuals can build resilience by learning to manage stress and adversity more effectively.

Acceptance and Commitment Therapy (ACT): Acceptance and commitment therapy (ACT) is another therapeutic approach that encourages individuals to accept their thoughts and feelings rather than trying to avoid or control them. ACT promotes psychological flexibility by helping individuals focus on their values and commit to actions that align with those values, even in the face of difficulties (Hayes, Strosahl, & Wilson, 2011). This approach can enhance resilience by fostering a sense of purpose and reducing the impact of negative emotions.

Mindfulness-Based Stress Reduction (MBSR): Mindfulness-based stress reduction (MBSR) is a trademarked therapeutic program combining mindfulness meditation with stress management techniques. MBSR teaches individuals to stay present and non-judgmental in the face of stress, which can reduce emotional reactivity and improve resilience (Kabat-Zinn, 1990). Regular mindfulness practice through MBSR can lead to greater emotional balance and a more resilient mindset.

By building emotional resilience through coping strategies, gratitude practices, and therapeutic techniques, individuals can better navigate life's challenges and maintain mental and emotional well-being. These practices foster a positive and adaptable mindset, allowing for greater life satisfaction and the ability to thrive even under challenging circumstances.

Social Connections: The Importance of Community

Maintaining strong social connections is crucial for mental and emotional well-being, particularly as we age. Social interactions provide a sense of belonging, reduce the risk of mental health issues, and even contribute to physical health. This section will explore the benefits of social connections, offer tips for building a support network, suggest ways to stay connected digitally and encourage community engagement.

Benefits of Social Connections

Social connections play a vital role in our overall well-being. They provide emotional support, a sense of purpose, and opportunities for engagement, all of which contribute to a healthier, more fulfilling life.

Reduced Risk of Depression and Anxiety: Social connections are a protective factor against depression and anxiety. Regular interaction with friends, family, and community members can reduce feelings of loneliness and isolation, which are significant risk factors for mental health issues (Santini et al., 2015). Studies have shown that people with strong social ties are less likely to experience depression and anxiety, as these connections provide emotional support and a buffer against stress (Cacioppo, Hughes, Waite, Hawkley, & Thisted, 2006).

Enhanced Sense of Belonging: Being part of a community or social network enhances the sense of belonging, which is fundamental to emotional well-being. This sense of belonging helps individuals feel valued and connected, fostering a positive self-image and resilience in facing challenges (Baumeister & Leary, 1995). Whether through family, friends, or community groups, social connections provide the affirmation and support needed to navigate life's ups and downs.

Improved Physical Health: Besides mental and emotional benefits, social connections positively impact physical health. Research has found that individuals with strong social networks have lower rates of chronic illnesses, such as heart disease and hypertension, and are more likely to engage in health-promoting behaviors (Holt-Lunstad, Smith, & Layton, 2010). Social interactions can motivate individuals to stay active, eat healthily, and adhere to medical advice, contributing to longevity and well-being.

Building a Support Network

Creating and maintaining a support network is essential for accessing the benefits of social connections. A strong support network provides emotional support, practical assistance, and a sense of community.

Reconnecting with Old Friends: Reconnecting with old friends can reignite meaningful relationships and provide a sense of continuity and shared history. Reaching out to friends from different stages of life, whether through social media or by organizing a reunion, can strengthen your support network and enhance your social life (Doherty & Feeney, 2004). These connections often offer deep understanding and shared experiences that can be exceptionally comforting.

Joining Clubs or Groups: Joining clubs or groups that align with your interests is a great way to meet new people and build connections. Whether it's a book club, a gardening group, or a fitness class, shared activities provide a natural context for forming friendships and expanding your social circle (Putnam, 2000). These groups also offer a regular social outlet, which is vital for maintaining consistent social interactions.

Volunteering in the Community: Volunteering is a fulfilling way to give back to the community while building social connections. By volunteering, you can meet like-minded individuals, contribute to causes you care about, and develop a sense of purpose (Wilson & Musick, 1999). Volunteering benefits the community and enhances your well-being by fostering social ties and providing a sense of accomplishment.

Staying Connected Digitally

In today's digital age, staying connected doesn't always require physical proximity. Digital tools offer numerous ways to maintain and strengthen social connections, especially when in-person interactions are limited.

Video Calls with Family and Friends: Video calls are a powerful way to stay connected with family and friends, regardless of distance. Platforms like Zoom, Skype, or FaceTime allow for face-to-face interactions that help maintain close relationships and reduce feelings of isolation (Hollis et al., 2015). Regular video calls can keep you engaged in the lives of your loved ones, even when you can't be together in person.

Social Media Groups and Forums: Social media platforms offer a variety of groups and forums where you can connect with others who share your interests. These groups provide a space to exchange ideas, offer support, and build friendships, even with people you've never met (Ellison, Steinfield, & Lampe, 2007). Participating in online communities can be particularly valuable for maintaining social connections when in-person interactions are limited.

Online Interest Groups: Beyond social media, there are numerous online platforms dedicated to specific hobbies or interests, such as cooking, photography, or travel. Joining these online interest groups allows you to engage with others who share your passions, exchange tips, and even collaborate on projects (Wellman & Hampton, 1999). These digital communities can offer a sense of belonging and connection that is both meaningful and enjoyable.

Community Engagement

Engaging with your local community is an excellent way to build social connections, contribute to your community, and stay active.

Attending Local Cultural Events: Local cultural events, such as art exhibitions, theater performances, or music festivals, provide opportunities to engage with your community and meet new people. These events attract diverse attendees, making them a great place to expand your social circle and experience new things (Putnam, 2000). Regularly attending these events can help you stay connected to the cultural fabric of your community.

Participating in Community Classes: Community classes, such as cooking workshops, language courses, or exercise classes, offer a structured environment for learning new skills while building social connections. These classes provide opportunities for personal growth and allow you to meet others with similar interests (Putnam, 2000). Regular participation in community classes can lead to lasting friendships and a stronger sense of community involvement.

Joining Neighborhood Associations: Neighborhood associations are local groups that work to improve the quality of life in their communities. By joining a neighborhood association, you can contribute to community initiatives, stay informed about local issues, and connect with your neighbors (Larsen et al., 2004). Being involved in these associations fosters a sense of belonging and gives you a voice in shaping your local environment.

Maintaining strong social connections through face-to-face interactions or digital means can enhance your mental and emotional well-being, improve your physical health, and enjoy a greater sense of belonging. Engaging with your community and building a robust support network are essential to creating a fulfilling and connected life.

Combatting Loneliness: Staying Socially Engaged

Loneliness is a significant issue that can have profound effects on both mental and physical health. Understanding the nature of loneliness, identifying its sources, and implementing effective strategies to stay socially engaged and connected are essential. This section will explore the impact of loneliness, help readers identify its sources, provide strategies to combat it, and discuss when to seek professional support.

Understanding Loneliness

Loneliness is feeling socially isolated or disconnected from others, even when not physically alone. It is a subjective experience that can vary in intensity and duration, but its impact on health is universally significant.

Emotional and Physical Consequences: Loneliness can lead to a range of emotional consequences, including feelings of sadness, anxiety, and a sense of emptiness. Over time, these feelings can contribute to the development of more severe mental health issues, such as depression (Cacioppo & Cacioppo, 2018). Physically, loneliness may cause a variety of adverse health outcomes, including increased inflammation, higher blood pressure, and weakened immune function (Hawkley & Cacioppo, 2010). Chronic loneliness can also lead to unhealthy behaviors, such as poor diet, lack of exercise, and substance abuse, further exacerbating its impact on physical health.

Increased Risk of Chronic Diseases: Research has shown that loneliness significantly increases the risk of developing chronic diseases. It is associated with a higher incidence of heart disease, stroke, and type 2 diabetes (Valtorta et al., 2016). The stress and anxiety that often accompany loneliness can lead to long-term wear and tear on the body, making individuals more susceptible to these conditions. Additionally, loneliness is as harmful as smoking or obesity in terms of its impact on health (Holt-Lunstad et al., 2015).

Impact on Mental Health: Loneliness is a significant risk factor for mental health disorders, particularly depression and anxiety. The lack of social interaction and meaningful connections can lead to feelings of worthlessness, hopelessness, and a diminished sense of purpose (Perlman & Peplau, 1981). Over time, chronic loneliness can erode self-esteem and make it difficult to engage in social activities, creating a vicious cycle that reinforces feelings of isolation.

Identifying Sources of Loneliness

Understanding the root causes of loneliness is essential for addressing it effectively. Loneliness can stem from various sources, and identifying these can help develop targeted strategies to overcome it.

Life Transitions (e.g., Retirement, Loss of a Spouse): Significant life transitions, like retirement, the loss of a spouse, or moving to a new location, are familiar sources of loneliness. These events often disrupt established social networks and routines, leaving individuals disconnected and alone (Victor et al., 2000). Adjusting to these changes can be challenging if they reduce social interaction.

Social Isolation: Social isolation, whether due to physical distance, health issues, or mobility limitations, can lead to loneliness. When individuals cannot participate in social activities or maintain regular contact with others, they may feel increasingly isolated (Cornwell & Waite, 2009). This isolation can be particularly pronounced in older adults or those living alone, who may have fewer opportunities for social engagement.

Lack of Meaningful Connections: Social interactions are not consistent enough to prevent loneliness; the quality of these interactions also matters. A lack of meaningful connections—relationships that provide emotional support, understanding, and a sense of belonging—can contribute to feelings of loneliness (Pinquart & Sörensen, 2001). Superficial or infrequent interactions may not fulfill the need for deep, meaningful connections, leaving individuals feeling lonely even in the presence of others.

Strategies to Combat Loneliness

Combating loneliness requires proactive steps to increase social engagement and build meaningful connections. Here are some practical strategies to help reduce feelings of loneliness:

Engaging in Group Activities: Participating in group activities, such as exercise classes, hobby groups, or community events, provides opportunities to meet new people and form connections. Group settings offer a sense of community and shared purpose, which can help alleviate loneliness (Haslam et al., 2016). Whether joining a book club, attending a fitness class, or participating in a local charity event, engaging with others in a group setting can provide social interaction and a sense of belonging.

Volunteering: Volunteering is an excellent way to combat loneliness by giving back to the community and building social connections. Volunteering offers a sense of purpose and fulfillment, which can counteract isolation and loneliness (Piliavin & Siegl, 2007). Additionally, volunteering often involves working with others, providing opportunities to form new friendships, and strengthening social networks.

Adopting a Pet: Adopting a pet can effectively combat loneliness for those who live alone. Pets provide companionship, unconditional love, and a sense of responsibility, all of which can reduce feelings of loneliness (McConnell et al., 2011). Caring for a pet can also encourage physical activity and social interaction, such as walking a dog or participating in pet-related events.

Starting a New Hobby: Starting a new hobby can provide both personal fulfillment and opportunities for social engagement. Hobbies that involve group participation, such as joining a cooking class, learning a new language, or taking up a sport, can help you meet like-minded individuals and form new connections (Perese & Wolf, 2005). Even solo hobbies can provide a sense of accomplishment and structure, alleviating feelings of loneliness.

Professional Support

In some cases, loneliness may persist despite efforts to stay socially engaged. When loneliness becomes overwhelming or begins to affect mental health, it may be necessary to seek professional support.

Speaking with a Therapist: Therapy can provide a safe space to explore feelings of loneliness and develop strategies for building connections. Cognitive-behavioral therapy (CBT) and other therapeutic approaches can help individuals change negative thought patterns and behaviors contributing to loneliness (Masi et al., 2011). A therapist can also provide support and guidance in navigating life transitions that may contribute to loneliness.

Joining Support Groups: Support groups offer a space for individuals to share their experiences and connect with others who are going through similar challenges. These groups can provide emotional support and practical advice, helping participants feel less alone (Yalom & Leszcz, 2005). Whether in-person or online, support groups can be a valuable resource for those struggling with loneliness.

Utilizing Helplines and Counseling Services: Helplines and counseling services provide immediate support for those experiencing loneliness. Many organizations offer free or low-cost counseling services, both in-person and via phone or online. These services can provide a lifeline for individuals needing immediate support or not ready to seek in-person therapy (Mann et al., 2004).

By understanding loneliness, identifying its sources, and implementing strategies to combat it, individuals can reduce feelings of isolation and enhance their social connections. Professional support can also be valuable for those needing additional help overcoming loneliness and building a more connected and fulfilling life.

Creativity and Aging: Engaging in Artistic Pursuits

Engaging in creative activities is a source of joy and fulfillment and offers significant mental and emotional benefits, particularly as we age. Whether painting, writing, crafting, or playing music, these activities stimulate the mind, reduce stress, and foster a sense of accomplishment. This section will explore the benefits of creativity, suggest various artistic activities, offer tips for finding inspiration, and encourage readers to showcase their creative work.

Benefits of Creativity

Creativity is a powerful tool for enhancing mental and emotional well-being. Engaging in creative pursuits provides numerous benefits that contribute to a healthier, more fulfilling life.

Enhanced Cognitive Function: Creative activities engage different brain areas, helping maintain and improve cognitive function as we age. Activities like painting, writing, and playing music require problem-solving, critical thinking, and memory, stimulating the brain and promoting neuroplasticity (Cohen, 2006). Studies have shown that engaging in creative activities can delay the onset of cognitive decline and help maintain mental sharpness in older adults (Flood & Phillips, 2007). This mental stimulation is crucial for keeping the brain active and healthy.

Reduced Stress and Anxiety: Creativity is an effective outlet for expressing emotions and reducing stress. Engaging in artistic activities allows individuals to focus on the present moment, providing a form of mindfulness that can reduce anxiety and promote relaxation (Sandmire et al., 2012). Art, writing, or music can be therapeutic, channeling emotions and releasing tension. This stress reduction improves mental and physical health by lowering blood pressure and boosting the immune system.

Increased Sense of Accomplishment: Completing a creative project, whether a painting, a poem, or music, brings a strong sense of accomplishment and pride. This feeling of achievement can boost self-esteem and provide a sense of purpose, which is particularly important as we age (Reynolds, 2010). Engaging in creative activities also offers opportunities for personal growth and self-expression, allowing individuals to explore new aspects of their identity and capabilities.

Exploring Artistic Activities

There are countless ways to engage in creative activities, each offering benefits and joys. Here are some suggestions for artistic pursuits that can be both enjoyable and beneficial.

Painting and Drawing: Painting and drawing are classic forms of artistic expression that allow individuals to explore their creativity through color, shape, and texture. These activities improve hand-eye coordination, focus, and fine motor skills while providing a relaxing and meditative experience (Stuckey & Nobel, 2010). Whether working with watercolors, oils, or simply sketching with a pencil, painting, and drawing can be profoundly satisfying and offer endless possibilities for creative exploration.

Writing (e.g., Poetry, Journaling): Writing is a versatile and accessible form of creativity that can take many forms, from poetry and journaling to short stories and memoirs. Writing allows individuals to express their thoughts, emotions, and experiences, providing a creative outlet and a way to process and reflect on life's events (Pennebaker, 1997). Writing can help improve cognitive function, enhance emotional well-being, and provide a lasting record of your creative journey, whether crafting poems or keeping a daily journal.

Crafting (e.g., Knitting, Scrapbooking): Crafting encompasses various activities, such as knitting, scrapbooking, quilting, and more. These activities allow creative expression and improve dexterity and concentration (Sullivan & Heid, 2017). Crafting can also be a social activity, providing opportunities to connect with others through shared interests. The tangible results of crafting projects—whether a knitted scarf or a scrapbook—offer a sense of accomplishment and can be cherished as handmade keepsakes.

Music (e.g., Playing an Instrument, Singing): Music is a powerful form of creativity that engages the mind and body. Playing an instrument or singing involves coordination, rhythm, and memory, all contributing to cognitive health (Wan & Schlaug, 2010). Music also has emotional benefits, such as expressing feelings and connecting with others. Whether learning a new instrument or joining a choir, music can be an enriching and social activity that enriches your life.

Finding Inspiration

Inspiration fuels creativity, and finding it can sometimes be a challenge. Here are some tips for staying motivated and inspired in your creative pursuits.

Visiting Art Galleries and Museums: Art galleries and museums are treasure troves of inspiration, offering exposure to various artistic styles, techniques, and cultural expressions. Visiting these spaces can spark new ideas and provide fresh perspectives on your creative work (Smith, 2006). Whether inspired by a particular painting, sculpture, or exhibit, these visits can reignite your passion for creativity and encourage you to experiment with new approaches.

Reading Books on Creativity: Books on creativity offer valuable insights into the creative process and provide practical advice for overcoming creative blocks. Reading about the experiences of other artists, writers, or musicians can inspire you to try new techniques or explore different mediums (Tharp, 2003). Books on creativity can also offer exercises and prompts to help you stay motivated and engaged in your creative practice.

Joining Creative Groups or Classes: Joining a creative group or class provides structure, support, and a sense of community. Whether it's a local painting class, a writing workshop, or an online crafting group, participating in these activities allows you to share ideas, receive feedback, and stay motivated (Csikszentmihalyi, 1996). Creative groups also offer opportunities to learn new skills and techniques from others, further enriching your creative journey.

Showcasing Creativity

Sharing your creative work with others can be a fulfilling and empowering experience. It allows you to connect with others, receive feedback, and inspire those around you.

Participating in Local Art Shows: Local art shows provide a platform to showcase your work and connect with other artists and art enthusiasts. Whether you're displaying paintings, crafts, or photography, participating in these events can boost your confidence and provide valuable exposure (McCarthy et al., 2004). Art shows also offer opportunities to sell your work, share your creative journey, and gain recognition within your community.

Starting a Blog or Social Media Page: Starting a blog or social media page dedicated to your creative work allows you to share your projects with a broader audience. These platforms provide a space to document your creative process, share tips and techniques, and connect with other creatives (Poletti & Rak, 2014). Blogging or sharing on social media can also help you build a community of followers who appreciate and support your work.

Hosting Creative Meetups or Workshops: Hosting creative meetups or workshops is a way to bring people together to share and celebrate creativity. Whether you're teaching a craft, leading a writing workshop, or organizing a jam session, these events foster community and collaboration (Baker, 2012). Hosting events allows you to share your passion with others and inspire them to pursue their creative interests.

Engaging in creative activities offers numerous mental and emotional benefits, enhances cognitive function, reduces stress, and provides a sense of accomplishment. By exploring artistic pursuits, finding inspiration, and showcasing your work, you can enrich your life and stay mentally and emotionally vibrant as you age.

6

NAVIGATING LIFE TRANSITIONS

Thriving in Retirement: Finding New Purpose and Joy

Retirement is a significant life transition that brings both opportunities and challenges. While it marks the end of a career, it also opens the door to new possibilities for personal growth, exploration, and fulfillment. This chapter will explore how to embrace the emotional and psychological changes that come with retirement, identify new passions, stay engaged through volunteering, and create a fulfilling and balanced retirement plan.

Embracing the Change

Retirement often involves a complex mix of emotions and psychological adjustments. It can be a time of excitement and relief, but it may also bring feelings of loss, uncertainty, and the challenge of redefining one's identity.

Letting Go of Work Identity: For many people, their work is a significant part of their identity. Retirement requires letting go of this identity, which can be complex and emotional. Without the structure and purpose that work provides, retirees may struggle with feelings of loss and a diminished sense of self-worth (Wang, 2007). It's essential to recognize that this transition is standard and offers an opportunity to explore new aspects of your identity beyond your career.

Adjusting to a New Routine: Retirement often significantly changes daily routines. The structure provided by a work schedule vanishes, replaced by the freedom to organize time as you see fit. While this freedom can be liberating, it can also be overwhelming if not managed thoughtfully (Moen, 2003). Developing a new routine that balances relaxation with activities that bring joy and fulfillment is essential for a smooth transition into retirement.

Overcoming Feelings of Loss and Uncertainty: Feelings of loss and uncertainty can explode during the early stages of retirement. These feelings may stem from losing professional identity, social connections, or a sense of purpose (Kim & Moen, 2002). Acknowledging them and seeking support from friends, family, or a professional is essential. Engaging in new activities and setting personal goals can also help alleviate these feelings by providing a sense of direction and accomplishment.

Identifying New Passions

Retirement is an ideal time to explore new interests and passions ignored during your working years. Discovering these passions can lead to a more fulfilling and joyful retirement.

Passion Discovery Questionnaires: One effective way to identify new passions is by using passion discovery questionnaires. These tools help you reflect on your interests, values, and activities that bring you joy. You can uncover new areas of interest by answering questions about what excites you, what you've always wanted to try, and what you feel passionate about (Vallerand et al., 2003). These questionnaires can provide clarity and direction as you explore new pursuits in retirement.

Reflecting on Hobbies and Interests from Earlier in Life: Another way to identify new passions is by reflecting on hobbies and interests you enjoyed earlier in life but may have set aside due to career or family obligations. Retirement offers the perfect opportunity to revisit these activities and rediscover the joy they once brought (Clarke & Korotchenko, 2011). Whether painting, gardening, or playing a musical instrument, reconnecting with these pastimes can provide a renewed sense of purpose and fulfillment.

Trying Out New Activities and Classes: Exploring new activities and classes is a great way to discover interests you may not have considered. Many communities offer a variety of courses and workshops for retirees, ranging from art and music to fitness and technology. Trying different activities helps you discover new passions and keeps your mind active (Menec, 2003). The key is to stay open to new experiences and permit yourself to experiment.

Volunteering and Giving Back

Staying engaged and giving back to the community is a fulfilling way to spend your retirement years. Volunteering benefits others and enhances your well-being by providing a sense of purpose and connection.

Volunteering at Local Charities: Volunteering at local charities is a rewarding way to contribute to your community while staying active and engaged. Whether helping at a food bank, tutoring students, or working at an animal shelter, there are many opportunities to make a difference (Wilson, 2000). Volunteering allows you to use your skills and experience to help others, which can be incredibly fulfilling and rewarding.

Mentoring Younger Generations: Mentoring younger generations is another meaningful way to give back during retirement. Sharing your knowledge, skills, and life experiences with younger individuals can profoundly impact their lives (Kram & Hall, 1996). Whether through formal mentoring programs or informal relationships, mentoring provides an opportunity to stay connected, pass on valuable lessons, and contribute to the development of the next generation.

Participating in Community Service Projects: Community service projects offer a hands-on way to contribute to your local area. These projects range from neighborhood clean-ups and environmental conservation efforts to building homes or organizing community events (Morrow-Howell, 2010). Participating in these projects benefits the community and fosters social connections and a sense of belonging, which is essential for mental and emotional well-being in retirement.

Creating a Retirement Plan

A well-thought-out retirement plan is essential for ensuring a fulfilling and balanced retirement. This plan should include goals for personal growth, social engagement, and leisure activities.

Setting Daily and Weekly Goals: Setting daily and weekly goals helps provide structure and a sense of purpose in retirement. These goals can be as simple as walking daily, reading a book each week, or learning a new skill (Locke & Latham, 2002). Having goals to work towards gives each day direction and helps maintain a sense of accomplishment and satisfaction.

Balancing Leisure and Productive Activities: A balanced retirement plan includes leisure and productive activities. While relaxation and leisure are needed, it's also beneficial to engage in activities that challenge you and contribute to your growth (Csikszentmihalyi, 1997). This balance ensures that retirement is enjoyable and meaningful, providing relaxation and personal development opportunities.

Scheduling Social Activities: Social activities are vital to a fulfilling retirement. Scheduling regular social interactions, whether meeting friends for coffee, attending community events, or joining clubs, helps maintain social connections and prevents loneliness (Holt-Lunstad et al., 2010). A retirement plan that includes social activities ensures that you stay connected, engaged, and supported during this new phase of life.

You can find new purpose and joy in this exciting chapter of life by embracing the changes that come with retirement, identifying new passions, staying engaged through volunteering, and creating a balanced retirement plan.

The Empty Nest: Rediscovering Yourself

The transition to an "empty nest" is a significant life change many parents experience when their children leave home, whether for college, work or to start their own families. This period can be challenging and liberating, offering an opportunity for self-discovery and renewed focus on personal relationships and growth. This section will explore empty nest syndrome, how to reconnect with your partner, ways to pursue personal development and strategies for building a supportive network.

The Empty Nest Syndrome

Empty nest syndrome refers to the sadness, loss, and loneliness parents often experience when their children leave home. While it is a natural and expected life transition, it can still have a profound emotional impact.

Emotional Impact of Children Leaving Home: For many parents, their identity has been invested in their role as caregivers. When children leave home, parents may struggle with purposelessness or a loss of identity (Bouchard, 2014). This emotional shift can lead to feelings of grief, sadness, and anxiety as parents adjust to the absence of daily interactions with their children (Sherman & Lansford, 2015). Understanding that these feelings are normal and part of the transition process is the first step in coping with them.

Coping with Feelings of Loss and Loneliness: Coping with the emotional impact of an empty nest involves acknowledging the loss while finding ways to fill the void. Engaging in activities that provide a sense of purpose, such as volunteering, pursuing hobbies, or spending time with friends, can help alleviate loneliness (Mitchell & Lovegreen, 2009). It's also essential to allow yourself to grieve and to seek support from others who have gone through similar experiences.

Adjusting to a Quieter Household: The transition to a quieter household can be jarring for parents who are used to the constant activity and noise of having children at home. This change can initially feel like a loss, but it also presents an opportunity to create a more peaceful and reflective environment (Hartocollis, 2005). Parents can use this time to focus on their needs, interests, and well-being, embracing the quiet as a chance to relax and recharge.

Reconnecting with Your Partner

The empty nest phase offers a unique opportunity for couples to reconnect and strengthen their relationship. With fewer daily responsibilities tied to parenting, couples can focus more on each other and explore new ways to enjoy their time together.

Planning Regular Date Nights: One of the simplest ways to reconnect with your partner is by planning regular date nights. These evenings provide an opportunity to spend quality time together, free from the distractions of daily life (Carr, 2004). Whether dining out, seeing a movie, or simply enjoying a walk together, regular date nights help maintain the bond and intimacy between partners.

Taking Up Shared Hobbies: Exploring shared hobbies is another effective way to reconnect. Activities such as gardening, cooking, or taking a dance class together can reignite the sense of partnership and shared enjoyment (Holmes & Johnson, 2009). Shared hobbies provide common ground for conversation and create opportunities for fun and adventure in the relationship.

Communicating Openly About Feelings and Needs: Open communication is crucial during this transitional phase. Couples must discuss their feelings about the empty nest and express their needs and expectations for this new chapter in their lives (Braithwaite & Baxter, 2006). By openly addressing concerns or fears, couples can support each other through the adjustment process and strengthen their emotional connection.

Pursuing Personal Growth

The empty nest phase is also ideal for personal growth and self-discovery. With more free time and fewer obligations, parents can explore new interests, develop new skills, and embark on adventures postponed during the child-rearing years.

Taking Up New Hobbies or Interests: This period offers the freedom to explore new hobbies or revive old interests. Whether learning a new language, trying out painting, or taking up a sport, engaging in activities that spark joy and curiosity can bring a renewed sense of purpose and fulfillment (Reynolds, 2010). Hobbies provide personal satisfaction and opportunities to meet new people and expand social circles.

Enrolling in Educational Courses: Lifelong learning is a powerful tool for personal growth. Enrolling in educational courses, whether online or in person, allows you to gain new knowledge, acquire new skills, and stay mentally active (Merriam & Kee, 2014). Continuing education can be intellectually stimulating and deeply rewarding whether you're interested in history, technology, art, or any other field.

Traveling and Exploring New Places: Traveling is another exciting way to embrace this new phase of life. Whether visiting new countries, exploring different cultures, or taking short trips within your region, travel broadens your horizons and provides fresh perspectives (McCabe & Johnson, 2013). Traveling during the empty nest phase can be particularly enriching, as it offers the flexibility to explore new destinations without the constraints of school schedules or work obligations.

Building a Support Network

Building and maintaining a solid support network is essential during the empty nest phase. Connecting with others provides emotional support, reduces feelings of isolation, and enhances overall well-being.

Joining Empty Nester Support Groups: Joining support groups specifically for empty nesters can provide a valuable space to share experiences, offer advice, and receive support from others going through similar transitions (Barrett, 2008). These groups, whether in person or online, offer a sense of community and understanding, helping to alleviate feelings of loneliness and uncertainty.

Staying Connected with Friends and Family: Maintaining solid relationships with friends and family is vital for emotional health during the empty nest phase. Regular communication, whether through phone calls, video chats, or in-person visits, helps keep these connections strong (Carstensen, 1992). Socializing with friends and family provides emotional support, a sense of belonging, and continued engagement with loved ones.

Participating in Community Activities: Community activities are another way to build a support network and stay socially connected. Whether volunteering, attending local events, or joining clubs and organizations, participating in community life fosters a sense of purpose and belonging (Menec, 2003). These activities also provide opportunities to meet new people, contribute to the community, and stay active and engaged.

While challenging, the empty nest phase also offers an opportunity to rediscover yourself, reconnect with your partner, and pursue personal growth. By embracing this life transition, building a solid support network, and exploring new interests, you can find joy and fulfillment in this new chapter of life.

Caring for Aging Parents: Balancing Your Needs and Theirs

Many individuals are responsible for caring for aging parents as they navigate midlife and beyond. While caregiving can be a rewarding experience, it also presents significant emotional and physical challenges. This section will explore the demands of caregiving, offer tips for effective communication with aging parents, suggest resources and support systems for caregivers, and emphasize the importance of self-care.

Understanding Caregiving

Caregiving for aging parents involves complex responsibilities that can significantly impact the caregiver's life. Understanding these demands is crucial for balancing caregiving duties and personal well-being.

Impact on Personal Time and Energy: The demands of caregiving can consume a significant amount of personal time and energy, often leading to feelings of exhaustion and overwhelm. Many caregivers juggle multiple responsibilities, including work, family, and individual needs, alongside their caregiving duties (Pinquart & Sörensen, 2007), reducing the time available for self-care, social activities, and other aspects of life vital for overall well-being.

Emotional Stress and Burnout: The emotional stress of caregiving can be profound. Caregivers often experience feelings of guilt, sadness, and anxiety as they watch their parents' health decline (Schulz & Sherwood, 2008). The constant worry and responsibility can lead to caregiver burnout, characterized by physical and emotional exhaustion, irritability, and helplessness. Recognizing and addressing the signs of burnout early is essential to prevent long-term emotional and physical health issues.

Balancing Caregiving with Other Responsibilities: Balancing caregiving with other responsibilities, such as a career, marriage, and parenting, can be particularly challenging. Caregivers may feel pulled in multiple directions, struggling to meet the needs of everyone who depends on them (Kim & Schulz, 2008). This balancing act requires careful time management, clear communication, and setting boundaries to meet all responsibilities without compromising the caregiver's health and well-being.

Effective Communication

Effective communication with aging parents is critical to navigating the challenges of caregiving. Open, empathetic communication helps build trust and ensures that the caregiver's and the parents' needs are addressed.

Discussing Sensitive Topics with Empathy: Discussing sensitive topics, such as health concerns, living arrangements, and end-of-life plans, requires empathy and patience. It's essential to approach these conversations respecting your parents' autonomy and dignity while being honest about their situation's realities (Pillemer & Suitor, 2006). Active listening and validating their feelings can help create a supportive environment where complex topics can be addressed constructively.

Setting Boundaries and Expectations: Setting boundaries and clear expectations is essential for maintaining a healthy caregiving relationship. It's important to communicate your limits and needs to avoid feeling overwhelmed or taken for granted (Fingerman et al., 2011). This includes setting specific times for caregiving tasks, discussing what you can and cannot do, and ensuring that your parents understand and respect these boundaries.

Involving Other Family Members in Discussions: Involving other family members in caregiving discussions can help distribute responsibilities and reduce the burden on one individual. Family meetings can effectively coordinate care, share concerns, and make collective decisions about your parents' needs (Hammer et al., 2005). Clear communication and cooperation among siblings and other relatives can foster a supportive network that benefits the caregiver and the aging parents.

Seeking Support

Caregivers do not have to navigate this journey alone. Resources and support systems are available to help caregivers manage their responsibilities and maintain their well-being.

Local Caregiver Support Groups: Joining a local caregiver support group allows one to connect with others in similar situations. These groups offer emotional support, practical advice, and a sense of community, which can be invaluable in reducing feelings of isolation and stress (Chien et al., 2011). Support groups often meet regularly and can provide a safe space to share experiences and learn from others.

Online Forums and Resources: For those who may not have access to local support groups, online forums and resources offer an alternative way to seek support. Websites dedicated to caregiving, such as AARP's caregiving site or the Family Caregiver Alliance, provide forums where caregivers can ask questions, share stories, and access a wealth of information on caregiving (Collins & Swartz, 2011). These online communities can be a lifeline for caregivers seeking advice or simply needing to connect with others who understand their challenges.

Professional Caregiving Services: In some cases, professional caregiving services may be necessary to provide the care your parents need. Hiring a professional caregiver can relieve some of the burden, allowing you to focus on other responsibilities or take much-needed breaks (Gaugler et al., 2005). Professional services can range from in-home care to adult day care centers, offering flexibility depending on your parents' needs and your availability.

Self-Care for Caregivers

Self-care is not a luxury for caregivers; it is a necessity. Taking care of your physical and emotional health ensures you can continue providing care without compromising your well-being.

Scheduling Regular Breaks and Time Off: Scheduling regular breaks and time off from caregiving duties is crucial for preventing burnout. Whether taking a few hours each week to pursue hobbies, spending time with friends, or simply relaxing, these breaks allow you to recharge and maintain your health (Zarit et al., 2010). If necessary, consider enlisting the help of other family members or professional caregivers to provide respite care.

Practicing Stress-Relief Techniques (e.g., Meditation): Incorporating stress-relief techniques, such as meditation, deep breathing exercises, or yoga, into your daily routine can help manage the emotional toll of caregiving. These practices promote relaxation, reduce anxiety, and improve overall mental health (Schulz et al., 2004). Even a few minutes of mindfulness or meditation each day can significantly improve your ability to cope with the stresses of caregiving.

Seeking Professional Counseling if Needed: If you find yourself feeling overwhelmed, depressed, or unable to manage the demands of caregiving, seeking professional counseling is a proactive step. A counselor or therapist can provide coping strategies, emotional support, and guidance on navigating caregiving challenges (Northouse et al., 2012). Professional support can be particularly helpful in managing complex emotions and preventing caregiver burnout.

Caring for aging parents requires balancing their needs with your own, communicating effectively, seeking support, and prioritizing self-care. By taking these steps, you can provide compassionate care while maintaining your health and well-being.

Grandparenting: Building Strong Bonds with Grandchildren

Being a grandparent is a unique and rewarding experience that allows you to build meaningful relationships with the next generation. Grandparents play a vital role in their grandchildren's lives, offering love, wisdom, and support. This section will explore grandparents' roles, suggest activities to strengthen bonds with grandchildren, provide tips for maintaining long-distance relationships, and discuss the importance of passing down family traditions.

Roles of Grandparents

Grandparents can fulfill several essential roles in their grandchildren's lives, each contributing to the child's emotional and social development.

Nurturer and Caregiver: As nurturers and caregivers, grandparents provide unconditional love, comfort, and security. This role often includes helping with day-to-day caregiving tasks, such as babysitting, providing meals, and offering a safe, loving environment (Mansson, 2013). Grandparents' involvement in these aspects of their grandchildren's lives helps to reinforce family bonds and provides children with an additional source of emotional support and stability.

Mentor and Teacher: Grandparents also serve as mentors and teachers, sharing their knowledge, life experiences, and values with their grandchildren. This role can involve helping with homework, teaching practical skills, or offering advice and guidance (King & Elder, 1995). By acting as mentors, grandparents contribute to their grandchildren's moral and intellectual development, helping them navigate life's challenges with wisdom and confidence.

Playmate and Companion: Besides their nurturing and mentoring roles, grandparents often act as playmates and companions, engaging in fun and creative activities with their grandchildren. This role allows grandparents to build strong emotional connections through shared experiences and laughter (Kennedy & Kennedy, 1993). Whether through games, storytelling, or outdoor adventures, being a playmate allows grandparents to bond with their grandchildren in a relaxed and joyful setting.

Activities to Bond

Engaging in activities together is one of the most effective ways for grandparents to strengthen their bonds with their grandchildren. These activities provide opportunities for connection, learning, and fun.

Storytelling and Reading Together: Storytelling and reading are timeless activities that entertain and educate. Grandparents can share life stories, pass down family history, or read books that spark imagination and curiosity (Zipes, 1995). These moments create a special connection between grandparent and grandchild, fostering a love of stories and learning.

Cooking and Baking Family Recipes: Cooking and baking offer an excellent opportunity to bond while passing down family traditions. Preparing family recipes allows grandchildren to learn about their cultural heritage and culinary traditions while enjoying the hands-on experience of creating something delicious (Dunifon et al., 2018). These kitchen activities are fun and allow grandparents to share their skills and create lasting memories.

Outdoor Adventures (e.g., Hiking, Fishing): Outdoor activities such as hiking, fishing, or gardening provide a chance to connect with nature and each other. These adventures encourage physical activity, exploration, and appreciation for the natural world (Freeman et al., 2018). Spending time outdoors together fosters a sense of adventure and shared discovery, helping to strengthen the bond between grandparent and grandchild.

Crafting and DIY Projects: Crafting and DIY projects are creative activities that grandparents and grandchildren can enjoy together. Whether making homemade gifts, scrapbooking, or building a birdhouse, these projects offer a way to express creativity and work collaboratively (Kotrla Topić & Ivanović, 2016). Crafting together results in tangible creations and deepens the connection through shared effort and artistic expression.

Maintaining Long-Distance Relationships

For grandparents who live far from their grandchildren, maintaining solid relationships requires creativity and consistent effort. Fortunately, there are many ways to stay connected across the miles.

Regular Video Calls and Phone Calls: Regular video calls and phone calls are essential for maintaining close relationships when distance separates you. These calls provide opportunities for face-to-face interaction, allowing grandparents to stay involved in their grandchildren's lives despite the distance (Hirsh-Pasek & Golinkoff, 2003). Scheduling regular calls helps establish a routine that grandchildren can look forward to, reinforcing the bond and keeping communication lines open.

Sending Letters and Care Packages: Sending letters and care packages adds a personal touch to long-distance relationships. Handwritten letters, postcards, or small gifts create tangible connections and remind grandchildren that they are loved and thought of (Bengtson, 2001). Care packages filled with favorite snacks, books, or crafts can be a delightful surprise that bridges the gap and strengthens the emotional connection.

Planning Visits and Vacations Together: Planning visits and vacations together provides quality time to strengthen personal relationships. Whether it's a weekend visit or a more extended vacation, these special occasions offer opportunities to create lasting memories and deepen the bond between grandparent and grandchild (Jang & Tang, 2016). Planning these visits together also builds anticipation and excitement, making the time spent together more meaningful.

Passing Down Traditions

Grandparents play an essential role in their grandchildren's lives by passing down family traditions and values. These traditions help maintain a sense of continuity and identity within the family.

Sharing Family History and Stories: Sharing family history and stories is a powerful way to connect grandchildren to their roots. By recounting tales of past generations, grandparents help children understand where they come from and instill a sense of pride and belonging (Hagestad, 1985). These stories can also teach important life lessons and values, contributing to the child's moral development.

Teaching Cultural Practices and Customs: Grandparents are often the keepers of cultural practices and customs; passing these down is a valuable way to preserve family heritage. Whether it's teaching traditional dances, songs, or rituals, these cultural practices help grandchildren connect with their cultural identity (Roberto & Skoglund, 1996). Engaging in these activities strengthens the family bond and ensures that these traditions are passed on to future generations.

Celebrating Holidays and Special Occasions Together: Celebrating holidays and special occasions together reinforces family traditions and creates cherished memories. Whether preparing a special holiday meal, decorating together or participating in religious rituals, these celebrations provide a sense of continuity and shared joy (Moorman & Stokes, 2016). Involving grandchildren in these traditions ensures they will carry these practices forward, keeping the family's legacy alive.

Grandparenting offers countless opportunities to build strong, loving bonds with grandchildren. By embracing various roles, engaging in meaningful activities, maintaining long-distance connections, and passing down traditions, grandparents can play a vital role in their grandchildren's lives, enriching their own lives and those of their grandchildren.

Downsizing: Simplifying Your Living Space

As you transition into retirement or a new phase of life, downsizing and simplifying your living space can offer numerous benefits, from reduced maintenance to increased flexibility. This section will explore the advantages of downsizing, provide tips for planning and organizing the process, offer practical advice on decluttering, and suggest ways to adjust to life in a smaller space.

Benefits of Downsizing

Downsizing involves moving to a smaller, more manageable living space, which can bring several significant benefits.

Reduced Maintenance and Upkeep: One of the primary advantages of downsizing is the reduction in the time, effort, and cost associated with maintaining a larger home. A smaller space generally means fewer rooms to clean, less yard work, and fewer repairs (Freeman, 2014). This reduction in maintenance tasks allows you to spend more time enjoying your retirement, pursuing hobbies, or traveling rather than being bogged down by household chores.

Lower Living Expenses: Downsizing can lead to lower living expenses, including reduced utility bills, property taxes, and insurance costs (Shearer & Moss, 2015). A smaller home typically requires less energy to heat and cool, and the overall cost of maintaining the property is generally lower. This benefit can provide greater financial security in retirement, allowing you to allocate more resources toward leisure activities, travel, or other priorities.

Increased Mobility and Flexibility: Moving to a smaller, more manageable home can improve your mobility and flexibility, especially if you choose a location that suits your lifestyle and needs better. For example, downsizing to a house in a walkable community, near public transportation, or in a retirement-friendly area can enhance your quality of life and make it easier to stay active and socially engaged (Kim & Lee, 2017). Additionally, a smaller home may allow for easier relocation in the future, should your needs or preferences change.

Planning the Downsizing Process

Downsizing is a significant transition that requires careful planning and organization. Here are some tips to help you navigate the process smoothly.

Creating a Downsizing Timeline: Creating a timeline for your downsizing process is essential for staying organized and reducing stress. Start by setting a target move date and then work backward to establish critical milestones, such as when to begin sorting through belongings, holding a garage sale, or scheduling movers (Johnson &

Gannon, 2014). A well-structured timeline will help you stay on track and ensure that you have enough time to make thoughtful decisions about what to keep, sell, donate, or discard.

Making a List of Essential Items: Before you begin the downsizing process, list essential items you cannot live without. These may include sentimental items, necessary furniture, and everyday household items (Morrison & Johnson, 2012). By focusing on what is truly important, you can make more informed decisions about what to keep and what to let go of, ensuring your new space feels comfortable and functional.

Deciding What to Sell, Donate, or Keep: Deciding what to sell, donate, or keep can be challenging, especially if you have accumulated a lifetime of belongings. To make this process easier, consider each item's value, utility, and emotional significance (Cherrier & Pon, 2012). Items still in good condition but no longer needed can be sold or donated, while those with sentimental value or practical use should be kept. This approach helps reduce clutter and ensures your new space reflects your current needs and lifestyle.

Organizing and Decluttering

Decluttering and organizing are crucial steps in the downsizing process. Here are some practical strategies to help you simplify your belongings.

Sorting Items by Category (e.g., Clothing, Books): One effective way to declutter is sorting items into categories, such as clothing, books, kitchenware, and personal mementos (Kondo, 2014). This method lets you focus on one category at a time, making the process more manageable and less overwhelming. As you sort through each category, consider whether each item adds value to your life and fits into your new space.

Using the "One-Year Rule" for Keeping Items: The "one-year rule" is a popular decluttering guideline that suggests keeping only those items that you have used within the past year (Millburn & Nicodemus, 2016). If an item has not been used in the last 12 months, you will likely no longer need it and can consider selling, donating, or discarding it. This rule helps streamline your belongings and ensures you only bring valuable and relevant items into your new home.

Donating or Selling Unused Items: As you declutter, consider donating or selling items that are still in good condition but no longer serve a purpose. Many charitable organizations accept donations of clothing, furniture, and household goods, providing a way to give back to the community while simplifying your space (Rivkin, 2013). Alternatively, holding a garage sale or selling items online can help you earn extra money that can be used for moving expenses or to enhance your new living space.

Adjusting to a Smaller Space

Adjusting to life in a smaller space can be a rewarding experience if approached with creativity and planning. Here are some tips for making the most of your new home.

Maximizing Storage Solutions: In a smaller space, efficient storage solutions are essential. Consider investing in multifunctional furniture, such as ottomans with hidden storage or beds with built-in drawers (Yanko, 2015). Vertical space with shelves and hooks can also help organize your belongings without wasting valuable floor space. Smart storage solutions will allow you to keep your home tidy and ensure everything has its place.

Creating Multifunctional Living Areas: In a smaller home, it's essential to develop multifunctional living areas that serve multiple purposes. For example, a dining area can double as a workspace, or a guest room can be designed to function as a home office when not in use (Mitchell, 2015). Creating flexible and adaptable spaces allows you to make the most of your square footage and maintain a comfortable and functional living environment.

Personalizing and Decorating the New Space: Personalizing and decorating your new space will help it feel like home. Even in a smaller space, you can express your style and personality through thoughtful decor choices, such as artwork, textiles, and color schemes (Innes, 2016). Incorporating personal touches, such as family photos or cherished mementos, can make your new home feel warm and inviting, helping you easily adjust to your new surroundings.

Downsizing offers numerous benefits, from reduced living expenses to increased flexibility, and can lead to a simpler, more manageable lifestyle. By carefully planning the downsizing process, organizing and decluttering your belongings, and making thoughtful adjustments to your new space, you can create a living environment that supports your needs and enhances your quality of life.

Financial Planning: Ensuring Stability in Your Later Years

Financial stability in your later years is essential for maintaining a comfortable and stress-free lifestyle. Careful financial planning becomes increasingly important as you enter retirement or approach your later years. This section will discuss the significance of financial planning, provide tips for effective budgeting and saving, offer tailored investment strategies, and suggest resources and tools to help you manage your finances effectively.

Importance of Financial Planning

Financial planning is crucial for ensuring you have the resources to maintain your lifestyle, manage expenses, and prepare for any unexpected challenges that may arise in your later years.

Managing Fixed Incomes: For many retirees, income comes from fixed sources such as Social Security, pensions, or retirement savings accounts. Managing a fixed income requires careful planning to ensure that your expenses do not exceed your income (Yuh & Hanna, 2010). Financial planning helps you create a sustainable budget that accounts for all your needs while allowing for some discretionary spending, ensuring that your fixed income can support your lifestyle.

Preparing for Unexpected Expenses: Unexpected expenses, such as medical emergencies, home repairs, or assisting family members, can quickly deplete your savings if you are not prepared. Financial planning allows you to build a buffer for these unexpected costs, reducing the risk of financial strain (Lusardi & Mitchell, 2014). Setting aside funds for emergencies allows you to navigate unforeseen challenges without compromising your financial stability.

Ensuring a Comfortable Lifestyle: A well-thought-out financial plan helps ensure that you can maintain a comfortable lifestyle throughout your retirement. Whether traveling, pursuing hobbies, or simply enjoying your daily routine without financial stress, having a clear financial strategy gives you the confidence to live your later years to the fullest (Wong & Hardy, 2009). This planning includes understanding your long-term financial needs and making informed decisions about how to allocate your resources.

Budgeting and Saving

Effective budgeting and saving are foundational components of a sound financial plan. Here are some tips to help you manage your finances wisely.

Creating a Retirement Budget: A detailed retirement budget is the first step in managing your finances effectively. Start by calculating your fixed income sources and list all your regular expenses, including housing, utilities, groceries, healthcare, and insurance (Hatcher, 2009). Don't forget to include discretionary spending, such as entertainment, travel, and dining out. A realistic budget helps you understand your financial limits and ensures that your spending aligns with your income.

Identifying Areas to Cut Expenses: Once you have a budget, look for areas where you can reduce expenses without sacrificing your quality of life, including downsizing your home, switching to a less expensive insurance plan, or cutting back on non-essential purchases (Blanchett, 2013). Minor adjustments in your spending habits can add up over time, helping you stretch your retirement savings further.

Setting Aside Emergency Funds: An emergency fund is essential for covering unexpected expenses without derailing your financial plan. Aim to set aside at least three to six months' living expenses in a liquid, easily accessible account (Garman & Forgue, 2011). This fund acts as a safety net, giving you peace of mind knowing you can handle financial surprises without having to dip into your long-term savings.

Investment Strategies

Investment strategies tailored to older adults focus on preserving capital while generating a steady income. Here are some approaches to consider.

Diversifying Investment Portfolios: Diversification is vital to managing risk in your investment portfolio. By spreading your investments across various asset classes, such as stocks, bonds, real estate, and cash equivalents, you reduce the impact of market volatility on your overall portfolio (Markowitz, 1952). Diversification helps protect your savings while allowing for growth potential, ensuring your portfolio remains resilient in different economic conditions.

Considering Low-Risk Investment Options: As you age, it's wise to shift towards lower-risk investment options, prioritizing capital preservation over high returns. Consider allocating a more significant portion of your portfolio to bonds, certificates of deposit (CDs), and other fixed-income securities that offer more stability and predictable returns (Campbell & Viceira, 2002). While these investments may not yield high returns, they provide a steady income stream with less risk to your principal.

Seeking Professional Financial Advice: Navigating the complexities of investment planning can be challenging, especially as you approach retirement. Consulting with a financial advisor specializing in retirement planning can provide valuable insights tailored to your situation (Finke et al., 2016). A professional can help you develop a personalized investment strategy, manage your portfolio, and make informed decisions that align with your financial goals.

Resources and Tools

Numerous resources and tools are available to help you manage your finances and ensure stability in your later years.

Online Budgeting Tools and Apps: Online budgeting tools and apps can simplify managing your finances. Tools like Mint, YNAB (You Need A Budget), and Personal Capital allow you to track your spending, monitor your investments, and create custom budgets from your smartphone or computer (Dunlop, 2017). These tools provide real-time insights into your financial situation, helping you stay on top of your budget and adjust as needed.

Financial Planning Workshops and Seminars: Attending financial planning workshops and seminars can provide valuable knowledge and skills for managing your finances. Many community centers, universities, and financial institutions offer seminars on retirement planning, estate planning, and investment strategies (Pfau, 2013). These events can help you better understand financial concepts and connect you with resources that support your financial well-being.

Consulting with a Financial Advisor: Finally, consulting with a financial advisor is a proactive step towards ensuring economic stability. A financial advisor can help you assess your financial situation, set realistic goals, and develop a comprehensive plan that addresses your retirement needs (Bengen, 1994). Whether you're just starting to plan for retirement or need help managing your investments, a financial advisor can provide personalized advice and guidance.

Financial planning is essential for ensuring stability and comfort in your later years. By creating a solid budget, saving wisely, adopting a thoughtful investment strategy, and utilizing available resources, you can secure your financial future and enjoy a fulfilling retirement.

7

SPIRITUAL WELLNESS AND FAITH

Daily Devotions: Strengthening Your Spiritual Life

Importance of Daily Devotions

Daily devotions are crucial in nurturing spiritual growth and fostering a deeper connection with one's faith. They serve as a dedicated time for reflection, prayer, and meditation, helping to ground individuals in their beliefs and providing a framework for daily life. For many, daily devotions are essential to spiritual well-being, offering peace and a renewed sense of purpose.

Creating a Routine for Spiritual Reflection: Establishing a daily devotional practice helps develop a routine for spiritual reflection, allowing individuals to engage with their faith regularly. This routine reinforces spiritual beliefs and creates a space for introspection and personal growth. Regular engagement with devotional materials can lead to a more disciplined and focused spiritual life, which is particularly important as one navigates the challenges and transitions of aging (Pargament, 2007).

Enhancing Personal Connection with Faith: Daily devotions also enhance personal connection with faith by fostering a deeper understanding of religious teachings and principles. Engaging with scripture or devotional readings allows individuals to fully explore their beliefs and apply these insights to their daily lives. This continuous engagement can strengthen one's relationship with the divine, providing comfort and guidance in times of uncertainty (Ellison & Fan, 2008).

Providing a Sense of Peace and Purpose: Regular devotional practice offers peace and purpose, which is invaluable in maintaining emotional and spiritual balance. Setting aside time each day for spiritual reflection can help mitigate stress, reduce anxiety, and promote well-being. Moreover, the themes often explored in devotional readings—such as gratitude, hope, and forgiveness—can inspire individuals to live with renewed purpose and direction (Koenig, 2002).

Choosing Devotional Materials

Selecting suitable devotional materials is critical to creating a meaningful and fulfilling practice. The materials should resonate personally and spiritually, offering insights that align with one's beliefs and life experiences.

Popular Daily Devotionals: One widely recommended book is *Jesus Calling* by Sarah Young. This book provides daily reflections that speak to the heart and soul. It is known for its comforting and uplifting messages, making it popular among those seeking to deepen their spiritual lives (Young, 2004).

Scriptures Relevant to Aging and Wisdom: Certain scriptures may offer particular resonance for those looking to focus on themes of aging and wisdom. For example, verses from the Psalms, Proverbs, and the Epistles often emphasize the value of wisdom, patience, and the strength found in faith—concepts that can be particularly meaningful during the later stages of life (Wright, 2010).

Inspirational Stories and Prayers: Besides traditional scriptures and devotionals, inspirational stories and prayers can enrich daily devotions. Stories of individuals who have faced adversity with faith and grace can offer powerful examples of resilience and hope. Including prayers that speak to one's personal experiences can make the devotional time more reflective and impactful (Thompson, 2012).

Creating a Devotional Routine

To fully benefit from daily devotions, it is essential to establish a consistent routine that allows for uninterrupted time for spiritual reflection.

Setting Aside a Specific Time Each Day: Consistency is essential in creating a meaningful devotional practice. It is helpful to set aside a specific time each day—whether in the morning, during lunch, or before bed—dedicated solely to devotional activities. This regularity helps make devotions a natural part of daily life, ensuring that spiritual reflection remains a priority (Willard, 2002).

Finding a Quiet, Comfortable Space: The environment in which one practices devotions can significantly influence the experience. A quiet, comfortable space free from distractions allows for deeper concentration and reflection. Whether it's a dedicated prayer corner in the home or a favorite chair by the window, the setting should foster a sense of peace and focus (Foster, 1998).

Using a Devotional Journal for Reflections: Keeping a devotional journal can enhance the devotional experience by providing a space to record thoughts, prayers, and reflections. Writing down insights and reflections can help clarify thoughts and reinforce the spiritual lessons learned during devotional time. Over time, this journal can become a cherished record of one's spiritual journey (Peterson, 2005).

Personal Testimonials

The benefits of daily devotions are often best illustrated through the experiences of those who have made this practice a central part of their lives.

Increased Sense of Peace and Direction: Many individuals who incorporate daily devotions into their routine report a heightened sense of peace and direction. For instance, Mary, a retiree struggling to transition from a busy career to a quieter lifestyle, found solace in her daily devotional time. This practice helped her rediscover her purpose and gave her the spiritual grounding she needed to navigate this life change gracefully (Glover, 2011).

Strengthened Faith and Resilience: Another powerful testament to the impact of daily devotions comes from John, who faced significant health challenges in his later years. Through daily scripture reading and prayer, he found the strength to endure his physical trials and maintained a robust and resilient faith. His devotional practice became a source of comfort and a reminder of the hope and peace found in his spiritual beliefs (Koenig, 2002).

By making daily devotions a part of one's life, individuals can strengthen their spiritual foundation, gain clarity and direction, and foster a deep connection with their faith. This practice offers a path to spiritual growth and well-being, providing peace and purpose in the journey through life.

Faith and Healing: Finding Comfort and Strength
The Connection Between Faith and Healing

Faith has long been recognized as a powerful force in healing, offering emotional and physical benefits. While modern medicine is crucial in treating illnesses, faith can significantly contribute to healing by providing comfort, reducing stress, and fostering resilience. The connection between faith and healing is well-documented, with numerous studies and personal testimonies highlighting how a solid spiritual foundation can lead to improved health outcomes.

Reduced Anxiety and Stress: One of the most immediate benefits of faith in the healing process is its ability to reduce anxiety and stress. Faith can offer peace and assurance when faced with illness or physical challenges, mitigating the fear and uncertainty that often accompany these experiences. Studies have shown that patients who rely on their faith during medical treatments tend to experience lower levels of anxiety and stress, which can positively influence their overall health and recovery (Koenig, 2012).

Enhanced Coping Mechanisms: Faith also enhances coping mechanisms, giving individuals the strength to endure difficult times. The belief in a higher power or the comfort derived from religious practices can empower individuals to face their challenges with a sense of purpose and hope. This coping strategy is fundamental in managing chronic illnesses or long-term health conditions, where emotional resilience is crucial for maintaining quality of life (Parga-ment, 2007).

Improved Overall Well-Being: The holistic benefits of faith extend beyond emotional support to encompass overall well-being. Faith can foster a positive outlook on life, encourage healthy lifestyle choices, and promote a sense of community and belonging—all of which contribute to better health outcomes. Individuals who actively engage in their faith are often more likely to experience greater life satisfaction and well-being, even in the face of physical ailments (Levin, 2001).

Scriptures and Prayers for Healing

Certain scriptures and prayers can offer profound reassurance for those seeking comfort and strength during illness. These spiritual texts provide hope and reinforce the belief in divine support and healing.

Healing Scriptures: The Bible contains numerous verses that speak directly to the theme of healing. For example, Psalm 147:3 states, "He heals the brokenhearted and binds up their wounds," offering comfort to those suffering emotionally or physically. Similarly, Isaiah 41:10 provides reassurance with the words, "Fear not, for I am with you; be not dismayed, for I am your God; I will strengthen you, I will help you, I will uphold you with my righteous right hand." These scriptures remind believers of God's presence and power in healing (Wright, 2010).

Prayers for Physical and Emotional Healing: In addition to scriptures, specific prayers can be a source of solace and strength. A prayer for physical healing might ask for God's intervention to restore health and vitality, while a prayer for emotional healing could seek peace and comfort during distress. These prayers often focus on surrendering one's worries to God and trusting in His plan, which can bring significant emotional relief (Peterson, 2005).

Affirmations of Faith and Strength: Affirmations are another valuable tool for reinforcing faith during difficult times. Statements such as "I am strong in the Lord and in the power of His might" (Ephesians 6:10) or "With God, all things are possible" (Matthew 19:26) can help individuals maintain a positive and faith-driven mindset, which is crucial for emotional and spiritual resilience (Thompson, 2012).

Faith-Based Healing Practices

Beyond prayer and scripture, several faith-based practices can support the healing process. These practices reinforce one's spiritual connection and provide a sense of community and support during times of need.

Participating in Prayer Groups: Prayer groups offer a collective space where individuals can pray for healing, share their concerns, and support one another. The power of communal prayer can be incredibly uplifting, as it fosters a sense of unity and shared faith. Research suggests that prayer groups can enhance feelings of support and connection, vital components of emotional healing (Levin, 2001).

Attending Healing Services: Many religious communities offer special healing services to provide spiritual support and promote physical and emotional recovery. These services often include praying for healing, laying on hands, and other rituals inviting divine intervention. Attending these services can reinforce one's faith and provide comfort during challenging times (Koenig, 2012).

Using Anointing Oils in Prayer: Anointing with oil is a traditional practice in many faiths, symbolizing the presence and power of the Holy Spirit in the healing process. Anointing oils can be a tangible reminder of God's healing presence when used during prayer. This practice can be significant for those comfortable with ritual and symbolism (Peterson, 2005).

Stories of Healing

The power of faith in the healing process is perhaps best illustrated through the personal stories of those who have experienced its effects firsthand. These testimonies offer hope and encouragement, demonstrating the profound impact that faith can have on physical and emotional recovery.

Miraculous Recoveries: There are countless stories of individuals who attribute their miraculous recoveries to the power of faith. For instance, Sarah, who was diagnosed with a terminal illness, experienced a complete recovery after her community held a series of prayer vigils. Her doctors could not explain the sudden improvement, leading Sarah to believe that her healing directly resulted from divine intervention (Koenig, 2012).

Emotional Healing and Peace: Faith can also bring about profound emotional healing besides physical healing. John, who struggled with severe anxiety following a personal loss, found peace and acceptance through daily prayer and scripture reading. Over time, his faith helped him to overcome his anxiety and find a renewed sense of purpose and direction in life (Thompson, 2012).

Strengthened Relationships with God: Many individuals report that their experiences of illness or suffering have led to a strengthened relationship with God. Mary, who endured a lengthy battle with cancer, found that her faith deepened significantly during her illness. She described her journey as spiritual growth, where each challenge brought her closer to God and reinforced her trust in His plan (Levin, 2001).

These stories highlight the profound connection between faith and healing, offering hope and encouragement to those seeking comfort and strength during difficult times.

Meditation and Prayer: Connecting with Your Inner Self

Meditation in Faith

Meditation has been a cornerstone of spiritual practice for centuries, serving to connect more deeply with one's faith and inner self. While meditation is often associated with mindfulness and relaxation, it takes on an even more profound significance within the context of faith. Integrating meditation into spiritual practice can enhance focus, deepen spiritual awareness, and help individuals find inner peace.

Enhancing Focus and Clarity: Meditation allows individuals to quiet the mind, which can help improve focus and clarity. Meditation provides a space to center thoughts and clear mental clutter in a world of distractions and constant noise. This clarity is cognitive and spiritual, enabling individuals to discern their spiritual path more clearly and stay aligned with their faith (Kabat-Zinn, 2003).

Deepening Spiritual Awareness: Through meditation, individuals can deepen their spiritual awareness, becoming more attuned to the presence of the divine in their lives. Meditation offers a way to listen to the quiet voice of spirituality that often gets drowned out by the busyness of daily life. This practice fosters a stronger connection with one's faith and helps internalize spiritual teachings deeper (Tisdell, 2003).

Finding Inner Peace: One of the most significant benefits of meditation within a faith context is cultivating inner peace. As individuals meditate on spiritual themes or scriptures, they often experience a profound sense of calm and reassurance. This peace is rooted in the understanding and acceptance of spiritual truths, providing comfort and stability in the face of life's challenges (Bourgeault, 2004).

Types of Meditation

Various types of meditation can be integrated with faith, each offering unique benefits and opportunities for spiritual growth. Here are a few that can be particularly powerful:

Contemplative Meditation: Contemplative meditation focuses on a specific thought, image, or concept related to one's faith, such as a passage from scripture, a religious symbol, or a theological concept. The goal is to immerse oneself in contemplation, allowing the chosen focus to permeate the mind and heart. This type of meditation can deepen understanding and bring new insights into spiritual beliefs (Keating, 2009).

Scripture Meditation: In scripture meditation, individuals reflect deeply on a particular verse or passage from sacred texts. This practice involves slowly reading a passage of scripture, allowing each word to resonate, and then meditating on its meaning and application in one's life. Scripture meditation is a way to internalize spiritual teachings and apply them to personal experiences and challenges (Peterson, 2005).

Guided Faith-Based Meditations: Guided meditations that

incorporate elements of faith can also be very effective. These meditations typically involve listening to a recording or following a leader who guides participants through a meditation that includes spiritual themes, prayers, or affirmations. Guided meditations can help individuals focus their thoughts and deepen their spiritual practice, especially if they are new to meditation (Foster, 1998).

Prayer Practices

Prayer is the cornerstone of spiritual life, serving as a direct line of communication with the divine. There are many ways to pray, each offering a unique path to deepening one's spiritual connection.

Structured Prayers: Structured prayers, such as *The Lord's Prayer*, provide a time-honored framework for communication with God. These prayers offer a familiar structure that can bring comfort and stability, especially during uncertainty or distress. The repetition of structured prayers can also help individuals focus their minds and open their hearts to spiritual guidance (Peterson, 2005).

Spontaneous, Personal Prayers: Unlike structured prayers, spontaneous prayers are more fluid and personal, reflecting the individual's immediate thoughts and feelings. These prayers allow for a more intimate and direct conversation with the divine, where one can express gratitude, seek guidance, or share concerns without following a set formula. This practice can make prayer feel more personal and connected to the realities of daily life (Foster, 1998).

Prayer Journaling: Prayer journaling is another powerful practice combining writing and prayer. Individuals can write their prayers, reflections, and spiritual insights in a prayer journal. This practice helps organize thoughts and feelings and records one's spiritual journey. Reviewing past entries can reveal patterns, growth, and answered prayers, further deepening one's faith (Thompson, 2012).

Creating a Sacred Space

The environment in which one practices meditation and prayer can significantly influence the depth and quality of the experience. Creating a sacred space dedicated to these practices can help set the tone for spiritual reflection and connection.

Using Symbols of Faith: Incorporating symbols of faith, such as a cross, a prayer rug, or religious icons, can make the space feel sacred and spiritually resonant. These symbols are physical reminders of one's beliefs and can help focus the mind during meditation and prayer (Foster, 1998).

Incorporating Candles and Incense: Using candles and incense can enhance the atmosphere of a sacred space, adding a sensory dimension to the experience. The soft glow of candles and the gentle scent of incense can create a calming environment that encourages deep reflection and prayer (Peterson, 2005).

Ensuring a Quiet and Undisturbed Environment: Finally, ensuring that the space is quiet and free from interruptions is essential. You might choose a time when the household is calm or set up in a secluded area of the home. The quiet environment allows for uninterrupted focus, making it easier to connect with one's inner self and the divine (Keating, 2009).

Community Worship: The Role of Spiritual Communities

Importance of Community Worship

Community worship is a fundamental aspect of spiritual life that offers numerous benefits, particularly as we navigate the challenges and joys of aging. Being part of a spiritual community can provide a sense of belonging, opportunities for shared faith experiences, and the chance to engage in collective worship and service. These elements contribute to a richer, more fulfilling spiritual journey.

Sense of Belonging and Support: One of the most significant benefits of participating in a spiritual community is the sense of belonging it fosters. Being part of a group that shares similar beliefs and values can create a strong support network, which is particularly important during times of personal or spiritual struggle. This sense of belonging helps individuals connect to something larger than themselves, providing comfort and reassurance (Putnam, 2000).

Shared Faith Experiences: Engaging in community worship allows individuals to share their faith experiences with others, which can deepen their understanding and commitment to their beliefs.

These shared experiences—whether through prayer, song, or communal rituals—reinforce spiritual teachings and offer a sense of solidarity among members. Sharing faith in a communal setting can also lead to spiritual growth as individuals learn from each other's insights and experiences (Ammerman, 2014).

Opportunities for Collective Worship and Service: Community worship provides opportunities for collective worship, where the combined spiritual energy of the group can enhance individual experiences. Collective worship, such as attending services or participating in communal prayers, allows individuals to express their faith in a supportive and encouraging environment. Additionally, spiritual communities often engage in service projects that reflect their faith's teachings, offering members the chance to live out their values through acts of kindness and service to others (Wuthnow, 1994).

Finding a Spiritual Community

Finding the right fit can be a profoundly gratifying process for those seeking to join a spiritual community. Here are some tips to help you find and connect with a spiritual community that aligns with your beliefs and values.

Visiting Local Places of Worship: One of the best ways to find a spiritual community is by visiting local places of worship. Attending services can give you a sense of the community's atmosphere, values, and practices, whether a church, synagogue, mosque, or temple. Take the time to explore different options to see which community resonates with you the most (Ellison & George, 1994).

Participating in Community Events: Many spiritual communities host events outside regular worship services, such as social gatherings, charity events, or educational programs. Participating in these events can provide a more informal way to get to know the community and its members. These events often introduce the community's culture and values, helping you decide if it fits you (Putnam, 2000).

Engaging in Online Faith Communities: In today's digital age, many spiritual communities extend their reach online, offering virtual services, discussion forums, and social media groups. Engaging with online faith communities can be particularly beneficial for those with mobility issues or who prefer connecting from home. These online spaces can provide spiritual support and a sense of community, even from a distance (Campbell & Törsleff, 2017).

Active Participation

Once you've found a spiritual community, actively participating can enrich your spiritual life and strengthen your connections with other members.

Joining Worship Services and Prayer Meetings: Regularly attending worship services and prayer meetings is foundational to participating in a spiritual community. These gatherings provide structured opportunities to engage with your faith, receive spiritual guidance, and connect with others. Consistent attendance can help reinforce your spiritual practice and build relationships within the community (Wuthnow, 1994).

Volunteering for Community Service Projects: Many spiritual communities are involved in service projects supporting their members and the broader community. Volunteering for these projects is a meaningful way to live out your faith through action. Whether helping at a food bank, participating in a community clean-up, or supporting local charities, these activities allow you to make a positive impact while strengthening your connection to your faith community (Ammerman, 2014).

Participating in Study Groups and Classes: Joining study groups or educational classes offered by your spiritual community can deepen your understanding of your faith and its teachings. These groups often provide a space for discussion, reflection, and learning, allowing you to explore spiritual topics in greater depth. Participating in these activities can also help you build closer relationships with other members who share your interests and commitment to spiritual growth (Putnam, 2000).

Stories of Community Impact

The value of spiritual communities is often best understood through the personal stories of those who have found support, joy, and purpose. These testimonials highlight community worship's profound impact on individuals' lives.

Enhanced Sense of Purpose: For many, joining a spiritual community has provided a renewed sense of purpose. Take, for example, Maria, who felt isolated after retiring and moving to a new city. She joined a local church and found spiritual guidance and opportunities to volunteer and engage with others. Through her involvement, Maria discovered a new purpose in supporting her community and deepening her faith (Ammerman, 2014).

Strengthened Faith Through Communal Activities: Joshua, a long-time synagogue member, shared how participating in communal prayers and study groups has strengthened his faith. The collective worship experiences, combined with the shared wisdom of his fellow members, have deepened his understanding and commitment to his spiritual journey. John credits his community with helping him navigate personal challenges and maintain a strong faith (Ellison & George, 1994).

Lifelong Friendships and Connections: Many individuals find that spiritual communities are a source of lifelong friendships and connections. Sarah, who joined a mosque after moving to a new country, found that the relationships she built within the community were instrumental in helping her adjust to her new environment. The shared faith and mutual support she experienced created bonds that have lasted for years, providing her with a sense of belonging and continuity (Campbell & Törsleff, 2017).

Being part of a spiritual community offers countless benefits, from a deepened faith to forming meaningful connections. Whether through worship, service, or study, actively engaging in a spiritual community can significantly enrich your spiritual life and provide support and joy throughout your journey.

Spiritual Practices: Incorporating Faith into Daily Life

Integrating Faith into Everyday Activities

Incorporating faith into daily routines is a powerful way to deepen spiritual practice and maintain a constant connection with the divine. By integrating spiritual practices into everyday activities, individuals can transform mundane tasks into meaningful rituals, reinforcing their beliefs and providing spiritual nourishment throughout the day.

Morning and Evening Prayers: Starting and ending the day with prayer is a foundational practice for many people of faith. Morning prayers can set a positive tone for the day, offering guidance and strength to face the challenges ahead. Evening prayers allow one to reflect on the day's events, express gratitude, and seek peace before rest. These prayers need not be lengthy; even a few moments of sincere reflection can significantly impact one's spiritual well-being (Koenig, 2012).

Blessing Meals and Family Members: Blessing meals and family members is another way to weave faith into daily life. Saying a blessing before meals is a simple yet profound act that acknowledges the sustenance provided by the divine and expresses gratitude for the food. Similarly, offering blessings to family members through words or gestures reinforces spiritual bonds and fosters a sense of unity and love within the household (Peterson, 2005).

Practicing Gratitude and Mindfulness: Gratitude and mindfulness are essential to a spiritually enriched life. Practicing gratitude involves regularly acknowledging the blessings and positive aspects of one's life through silent reflection, prayer, or journaling. On the other hand, mindfulness is about being fully present in each moment and recognizing the divine in all things. Together, these practices cultivate a deeper awareness of the spiritual dimension in everyday life (Thompson, 2012).

Faith-Based Rituals

In addition to integrating faith into daily activities, simple faith-based rituals can be powerful reminders of one's spiritual journey. These rituals are not only acts of devotion but also opportunities to pause and reconnect with the divine presence.

Lighting a Candle for Prayer: Lighting a candle during prayer is a symbolic act representing the light of faith and the presence of the divine. This simple ritual can be performed at any time of the day, creating a sacred space for prayer and reflection. The soft glow of the candle can help focus the mind and elevate the spirit, making the prayer experience more profound (Foster, 1998).

Using Prayer Beads or Rosaries: Prayer beads or rosaries are traditional tools used in many faiths to guide prayer and meditation. Each bead or knot on the rosary represents a prayer, helping the individual stay focused and centered during their spiritual practice. This tactile element adds a sensory dimension to worship, making it a more immersive and contemplative experience (Keating, 2009).

Reading Daily Scripture Passages: Reading scripture daily is a practice that nourishes the soul and provides spiritual guidance. By setting aside time daily to read a passage from sacred texts, individuals can gain insights, find comfort, and strengthen their faith. Whether reading a single verse or a longer chapter, this practice helps keep spiritual teachings at the forefront of one's mind throughout the day (Wright, 2010).

Spiritual Acts of Kindness

Faith is often expressed through actions, and practicing acts of kindness is a powerful way to live out one's beliefs. These acts benefit others and reinforce the spiritual principles of compassion, generosity, and love.

Volunteering at Local Charities: Volunteering is a direct way to practice faith through service. By dedicating time to help those in need, whether through local charities, food banks, or community organizations, individuals can make a tangible difference in their communities while fulfilling the spiritual call to serve others. Volunteering also fosters a sense of connection and purpose, vital components of a spiritually fulfilling life (Ammerman, 2014).

Helping Neighbors and Friends: Acts of kindness don't always have to be part of organized efforts; they can be as simple as helping a neighbor with a task or offering support to a friend in need. These small, everyday acts of kindness are expressions of faith that strengthen relationships and build community. They remind us that spirituality is about personal devotion and how we interact with and care for those around us (Putnam, 2000).

Donating to Causes They Believe In: Financial donations to causes that align with one's spiritual values are another way to practice faith through action. Whether supporting a local church, funding a charitable organization, or contributing to a global humanitarian effort, these donations are expressions of generosity and compassion. They allow individuals to extend their spiritual influence beyond their immediate surroundings, positively impacting a broader scale (Ellison & George, 1994).

Documenting Spiritual Journey

Documenting one's spiritual journey is a valuable practice that allows for reflection, growth, and a deeper understanding of one's faith. By keeping a record of spiritual experiences, prayers, and insights, individuals can track their spiritual progress and remain focused on their spiritual goals.

Keeping a Faith Journal: A faith journal is a personal space where individuals can record their prayers, reflections, and spiritual experiences. Writing in a faith journal regularly encourages introspection and provides a tangible record of one's spiritual journey. Over time, this journal can reveal patterns, highlight growth areas, and serve as a source of inspiration during difficult times (Thompson, 2012).

Reflecting on Spiritual Growth and Experiences: Reflection is crucial to spiritual development. Reflecting on past experiences, challenges, and successes allows individuals to gain insights into their spiritual journey and understand how they have grown in their faith. Reflection can be done through journaling, meditation, or discussion with a spiritual mentor (Keating, 2009).

Setting Spiritual Goals and Intentions: Setting spiritual goals and intentions is a proactive way to guide spiritual development. These goals might include deepening prayer practices, learning more about sacred texts, or committing to acts of service. By setting specific, achievable goals, individuals can stay motivated and focused on their spiritual growth, ensuring their faith continues to evolve and flourish (Foster, 1998).

Leaving a Legacy: Making a Positive Impact

Understanding Spiritual Legacy

A spiritual legacy is the lasting impact of one's faith, values, and actions on future generations. It is the imprint left on the hearts and minds of family, friends, and community members long after we are gone. Understanding and intentionally cultivating a spiritual legacy can provide a sense of fulfillment and purpose, knowing that our lives will continue to influence and inspire others.

Impact on Family and Community: The most immediate recipients of a spiritual legacy are often family members and close friends. By consistently living out one's faith and values, individuals can shape the beliefs and behaviors of those around them. A spiritual legacy can provide guidance, comfort, and inspiration, offering a moral and ethical framework that helps loved ones navigate life's challenges (Koenig, 2012). Beyond the family, this legacy can extend to the broader community, influencing collective values and contributing to a culture of compassion, integrity, and service.

Continuation of Faith and Values: A spiritual legacy ensures that one's faith and values are passed down through generations, maintaining a continuity of belief and practice. This transmission of spiritual wisdom can help younger generations find meaning and direction in their lives, especially during difficult times. It also reinforces the idea that faith is not just a personal journey but a shared experience that connects individuals across time and space (Foster, 1998).

Sense of Fulfillment and Purpose: Knowing that one's life has positively impacted others can bring profound fulfillment. By consciously shaping a spiritual legacy, individuals can find purpose in their later years, contributing to something greater than themselves. This sense of purpose can enhance emotional and spiritual well-being, providing a more profound sense of satisfaction and peace as one approaches the end of life (Thompson, 2012).

Documenting Your Legacy

Documenting and sharing one's spiritual legacy is a meaningful way to ensure it endures. Various methods exist for capturing and preserving the lessons, stories, and values that have defined one's spiritual journey.

Writing Memoirs or Letters: Writing memoirs or personal letters is a powerful way to share your spiritual experiences, beliefs, and wisdom. These writings can be a gift to future generations, offering them insights into your faith and values. Whether it's a detailed memoir or a series of letters, this documentation lets you articulate the lessons you've learned and the principles you hold dear (Peterson, 2005). Such writings can guide your descendants, helping them understand their roots and draw strength from your experiences.

Creating a Family History Book: A family history book incorporating spiritual teachings and reflections can be an invaluable resource for future generations. This book can include genealogical information and stories of how faith has influenced your family's journey. By preserving these narratives, you provide a spiritual and historical context that helps future generations appreciate their heritage and understand the role of faith in their lives (Wright, 2010).

Recording Video Messages: In today's digital age, recording video messages is another effective way to document your spiritual legacy. These videos can be deeply personal, allowing you to speak directly to your loved ones and share your beliefs, hopes, and blessings. Video messages add a visual and emotional dimension that can be incredibly impactful, helping your legacy resonate more personally (Keating, 2009).

Teaching and Mentoring

Passing on faith and wisdom to younger generations is one of the most meaningful ways to build a spiritual legacy. By teaching and mentoring, you can directly influence the spiritual development of others, helping them grow in their faith and understanding.

Mentoring Youth in the Community: Mentoring young people in your community is a powerful way to impart spiritual wisdom. By building relationships with younger individuals, you can offer guidance, support, and encouragement, helping them navigate life's challenges with faith and integrity. Mentoring is not just about sharing knowledge; it's about being a positive role model who embodies the values and principles you wish to pass on (Putnam, 2000).

Leading Faith-Based Classes or Groups: Leading or participating in faith-based classes or study groups allows you to share your spiritual knowledge and insights with others. Whether it's a Bible study group, a prayer circle, or a discussion group on spiritual topics, these gatherings provide a platform for teaching and learning. Leading these groups can foster a deeper understanding of faith and create a supportive community for spiritual growth (Ammerman, 2014).

Sharing Personal Faith Stories and Experiences: Personal stories are powerful tools for teaching and inspiring others. Sharing your spiritual journey—the challenges you've faced, the lessons you've learned, and the faith that has sustained you—can profoundly impact those who hear them. These stories can provide inspiration and guidance, offering others the strength and hope they need to navigate their spiritual paths (Campbell & Törsleff, 2017).

Living a Legacy

A spiritual legacy is about what you leave behind and how you live each day. By living out your faith and values through your actions and choices, you can create a legacy that speaks louder than words.

Demonstrating Faith Through Daily Actions: One of the most effective ways to build a spiritual legacy is by consistently demonstrating your faith through your daily actions. Whether through acts of kindness, honesty in your dealings, or showing compassion to those in need, your actions reflect your beliefs. Living your faith authentically and openly sets an example for others to follow, showing them the power and importance of living according to one's values (Foster, 1998).

Supporting Community Initiatives: Actively supporting community initiatives that align with your faith is another way to live out your spiritual legacy. Whether volunteering at a local charity, participating in community outreach programs, or advocating for social justice, these actions demonstrate your commitment to living out your values in a tangible way. By engaging in these activities, you contribute to the well-being of your community and reinforce the principles you hold dear (Ammerman, 2014).

Leading by Example in Faith and Service: Leadership in faith and service is about setting an example for others. Whether within your family, church, or community, leading by example in how you practice your faith and serve others can inspire and guide those around you. This leadership is not about recognition or accolades; it's about living in a way that reflects your beliefs and encourages others to do the same (Koenig, 2012).

8

PRACTICAL SELF-CARE AND LIFESTYLE TIPS

Quick Self-Care Routines: Fitting Wellness into Busy Days

Importance of Quick Self-Care

In today's fast-paced world, finding time for self-care can be challenging, especially for those with busy schedules. However, even short self-care routines are vital for maintaining overall well-being. These quick, intentional moments of self-care can significantly impact your mental, emotional, and physical health.

Reducing Stress: Stress is a frequent experience, but regular self-care practices can help manage and mitigate its effects. Engaging in brief moments of relaxation or mindfulness throughout the day can lower cortisol levels, the body's primary stress hormone, leading to a calmer and more centered state of mind (McEwen, 2007).

Enhancing Mood: Self-care routines, even those that take just a few minutes, can boost mood and emotional resilience. Activities such as deep breathing or listening to music trigger the release of endorphins, the body's natural mood enhancers. These quick boosts can help maintain a positive outlook, even on the busiest days (Pressman et al., 2009).

Boosting Energy: Taking short breaks for self-care can also help replenish energy levels. Simple activities like stretching or drinking a glass of water can refresh both body and mind, allowing you to stay alert and focused throughout the day. Regularly incorporating these mini-breaks into your routine can prevent the afternoon energy slump and increase overall productivity (Puetz, Flowers, & O'Connor, 2008).

Preventing Burnout: Consistently neglecting self-care can lead to burnout, characterized by chronic stress, exhaustion, and emotional depletion. Integrating quick self-care routines into your daily schedule can prevent burnout before it starts, ensuring that you remain mentally and physically capable of handling life's demands (Maslach & Leiter, 2016).

Morning Self-Care Rituals

Starting the day with a positive and mindful routine sets the tone for the hours ahead. Morning self-care rituals don't have to be time-consuming; even a few minutes dedicated to self-care can make a significant difference.

5-Minute Meditation: Beginning the day with a short meditation session can help you cultivate mindfulness and focus. This practice involves sitting quietly, focusing on your breath, and allowing thoughts to come and go without judgment. Even just five minutes of meditation can reduce stress and improve concentration for the rest of the day (Zeidan et al., 2010).

Stretching Exercises: A quick stretching routine in the morning can wake up your muscles and improve circulation. Simple stretches, such as reaching for the sky, touching your toes, or performing gentle neck and shoulder rolls, can increase flexibility and reduce stiffness, helping you feel more energized and ready to tackle the day (Anderson & Burke, 2010).

Drinking a Glass of Warm Lemon Water: Starting the day with a glass of warm lemon water is a simple habit that can boost hydration and aid digestion. The vitamin C in lemons supports the immune system, while warm water helps stimulate the digestive tract, preparing your body for the day ahead (Ashurst, 2017).

Setting Daily Intentions: Setting positive intentions for the day can help you stay focused and motivated. This practice involves reflecting on what you want to achieve and how you want to feel, whether it's being more patient, staying positive, or completing specific tasks. Setting intentions creates a mental roadmap for the day, guiding your actions and decisions (Dweck, 2006).

Midday Pick-Me-Ups

The midday slump is an everyday experience, but a quick self-care activity can help you recharge and stay productive for the rest of the day. These small, rejuvenating practices can provide the boost you need to maintain energy and focus.

Quick Walk Around the Block: A brief walk outside can improve your energy levels and mental clarity. Physical activity increases blood flow to the brain, enhancing cognitive function, while exposure to natural light can improve mood and regulate your circadian rhythm (Hartig, Mang, & Evans, 1991).

Deep Breathing Exercises: Taking a few minutes to practice deep breathing can reduce stress and increase oxygen flow to your brain, helping you feel more alert and relaxed. Techniques such as diaphragmatic breathing or the 4-7-8 method effectively calm the mind and reduce tension (Jerath et al., 2006).

Listening to a Favorite Song: Music has a powerful effect on mood and energy levels. Listening to an upbeat or soothing song during a break can instantly lift your spirits and provide a mental reset. This simple act of self-care can help you return to your tasks with renewed focus and positivity (Thoma et al., 2013).

Evening Wind-Down

As the day comes to a close, winding down with a relaxing self-care routine is essential for preparing the body and mind for restful sleep. These evening practices can help you transition from the busyness of the day to a state of calm and relaxation.

Taking a Warm Bath: A warm bath is a classic way to relax and soothe tired muscles. The warm water helps lower your body temperature after you get out, signaling to your body that it's time to sleep. Adding Epsom salts or essential oils like lavender can enhance the experience, providing additional relaxation benefits (Nagai et al., 2000).

Reading a Book: Reading a few pages before bed can help you unwind and shift your focus away from the day's stresses. It's a mentally engaging yet calming activity that can prepare your mind for sleep. Choose something light and relaxing rather than a thriller that might keep you up late (Berkman et al., 2011).

Practicing Gratitude Journaling: Ending the day with a gratitude journal can help you reflect on the positive aspects of your day and cultivate a sense of contentment. Writing down a few things you're grateful for each evening can shift your focus from what went wrong to what went right, promoting a peaceful and positive mindset before bed (Emmons & McCullough, 2003).

Holistic Beauty: Natural Tips for Looking Your Best

Benefits of Holistic Beauty

Holistic beauty focuses on natural practices that enhance your appearance while promoting overall health and well-being. Unlike conventional beauty products, which often contain harsh chemicals, holistic beauty practices use gentle natural ingredients on the skin and body.

Fewer Chemicals and Side Effects: One of the main advantages of holistic beauty is reduced exposure to harmful chemicals. Conventional beauty products often contain synthetic ingredients like parabens, sulfates, and artificial fragrances, which can irritate the skin and cause long-term health issues (Guthrie et al., 2015). Opting for natural alternatives minimizes the risk of side effects, making maintaining healthy skin and hair easier.

Long-Term Skin Health: Natural beauty practices are often gentler on the skin and better suited for long-term use. Ingredients like coconut oil, aloe vera, and honey nourish the skin without clogging pores or causing irritation. These natural products work with the skin's natural processes, promoting hydration, healing, and regeneration, leading to healthier, more resilient skin over time (McCarty, 2012).

Environmental Benefits: Using natural beauty products also benefits the environment. Many synthetic ingredients in conventional beauty products are derived from non-renewable resources and can harm ecosystems when washed down the drain (Amberg & Fogarassy, 2019). By choosing natural, eco-friendly products, you contribute to environmental sustainability while caring for your beauty needs.

Natural Skincare Tips

Maintaining healthy, glowing skin doesn't require expensive products or complicated routines. Simple, natural ingredients can be incredibly effective in nurturing and protecting your skin.

Using Coconut Oil as a Moisturizer: Coconut oil is a versatile and natural moisturizer for the face and body. It is rich in fatty acids, which help to hydrate and protect the skin's barrier (Evangelista et al., 2014). Apply a small amount to clean the skin and massage it gently until absorbed. Its antimicrobial properties also make it worthwhile for soothing irritated skin and reducing the risk of infections.

Applying Aloe Vera for Soothing Irritated Skin: Aloe vera is a well-known natural remedy for soothing skin irritation, burns, and inflammation. Its anti-inflammatory properties help to calm redness and discomfort, making it an excellent choice for sensitive or sunburned skin (Surjushe, Vasani, & Saple, 2008). For best results, use pure aloe vera gel directly from the plant or choose a product with minimal additives.

Exfoliating with Oatmeal and Honey: Regular exfoliation helps remove dead skin cells and promotes a brighter, more even complexion. You can make a gentle, natural exfoliant by combining oatmeal and honey. Oatmeal is a mild exfoliant, while honey provides moisturizing and antibacterial benefits (Majewski, 2014). Mix the ingredients into a paste, apply to damp skin, and massage gently in circular motions before rinsing with warm water.

Hair Care with Natural Products

Healthy hair care can also be achieved through natural methods, using ingredients that nourish the hair without the harsh effects of chemicals.

Using Apple Cider Vinegar as a Hair Rinse: Apple cider vinegar (ACV) is an excellent natural hair rinse that helps balance the scalp's pH and removes product buildup, leaving hair shiny and soft (Fenton, 2012). To use, dilute one part ACV with two parts water and pour the mixture over your hair after shampooing. Rinse thoroughly with cool water to seal the hair cuticle and enhance shine.

Applying Coconut Oil for Deep Conditioning: Coconut oil is also beneficial for hair, providing deep conditioning that helps to repair damage, reduce frizz, and add shine (Rele & Mohile, 2003). For a deep conditioning treatment, warm a small amount of coconut oil in your hands and apply it to the ends of your hair, working your way up. Leave it on for at least 30 minutes or overnight for intense hydration, and then wash it out with shampoo.

Avoiding Heat Styling Tools: While styling tools like hairdryers, straighteners, and curling irons can create beautiful looks, frequent use can damage hair and lead to dryness and breakage. Opting for heat-free styling methods, such as braiding wet hair for waves or using foam rollers, can protect your hair's health and reduce the need for damaging heat (Aitken et al., 2007).

DIY Beauty Recipes

Creating your beauty products at home is a fun and cost-effective way to take control of what you put on your skin and hair. These simple DIY recipes use natural ingredients that you might already have in your kitchen.

Avocado Face Mask: Avocado is rich in healthy fats and vitamins that nourish and hydrate the skin. To make an avocado face mask, mash half an avocado and mix it with a tablespoon of honey. Apply the mixture to clean skin and leave it on for 15-20 minutes before rinsing with warm water. This mask helps to moisturize and rejuvenate the skin, leaving it soft and glowing (Nguyen et al., 2014).

Green Tea and Honey Toner: Green tea is packed with antioxidants, which help to protect the skin from environmental damage, while honey has antibacterial and moisturizing properties. To make a green tea and honey toner, brew a cup of green tea, let it cool, and mix in a teaspoon of honey. Apply the toner to your face using a cotton pad or spray bottle for a refreshing, hydrating boost (Lee et al., 2013).

Coffee Grounds Scrub: Coffee grounds are an excellent natural exfoliant that can help improve circulation and reduce the appearance of cellulite. To make a coffee scrub, mix used coffee grounds with a tablespoon of coconut oil and a teaspoon of sugar. Massage the mixture into damp skin in circular motions, focusing on areas where you want to improve skin texture. Rinse with warm water to reveal smooth, revitalized skin (Koo, 2013).

Travel Tips for Seniors: Exploring the World Safely

Planning Senior-Friendly Travel

Traveling can be an enriching experience at any age, but as we age, it's essential to consider certain factors that ensure trips are safe, comfortable, and enjoyable. Thoughtful planning can make a significant difference in how smoothly a journey unfolds.

Researching Senior-Friendly Destinations: When planning a trip, choosing destinations that are accommodating and accessible for seniors is critical. Many cities and countries now focus on making their attractions, transportation systems, and accommodations more senior-friendly (Rosenbloom & Stahl, 2003). Look for destinations that offer good public transportation, plenty of resting spots, and attractions that are not overly strenuous to explore.

Planning for Accessible Accommodations: Accessibility is crucial when choosing where to stay. Ensure your accommodations include elevators, ramps, and accessible bathrooms with grab bars (Ziegler, 2012). Selecting hotels or rental properties close to the places you plan to visit is also helpful to minimize travel time and effort.

Considering Travel Insurance: Travel insurance is essential for senior travelers. Policies that cover health emergencies, trip cancellations, and lost luggage can provide peace of mind (Rogers & Jarrett,

2007). Make sure to choose a plan that includes coverage for pre-existing conditions, a common concern for older adults.

Packing Essential Medications: Before traveling, ensure that you have enough of your prescribed medications for the entire trip, plus a few extra days in case of delays. Keep medicines in their original containers and carry a copy of your prescriptions and a note from your doctor explaining their necessity (Smith & Klein, 2009). Packaging a first aid kit with over-the-counter remedies for common issues such as headaches, allergies, or digestive problems is also advisable.

Health and Safety Tips

Maintaining health and safety during travel is paramount for senior travelers. Taking extra precautions can help avoid potential problems and ensure a pleasant trip.

Staying Hydrated: Dehydration can be a significant issue, especially during long flights or when spending time outdoors. Seniors should carry a reusable water bottle and drink fluids regularly throughout the day (Coyle, 2004). It's also a good idea to avoid alcohol and caffeine, which can contribute to dehydration.

Taking Regular Breaks: Whether walking through a city or visiting a museum, taking regular breaks is essential. Overexertion can lead to fatigue or injury, so listen to your body and rest when needed (Manini, 2010). Look for shaded areas, benches, or cafes where you can sit down, relax, and recharge.

Avoiding Overexertion: It's important to pace yourself when traveling. Plan activities with plenty of time in between, and avoid scheduling too many strenuous activities on the same day (Fried, 2010). Use mobility aids such as walking sticks or portable folding stools to help reduce strain.

Knowing Emergency Contact Information: Before departing, compile a list of emergency contacts, including local emergency numbers, your country's embassy or consulate, and contact information for friends or family members. Carry this list with you at all times, and ensure that someone at home knows your travel itinerary and how to reach you (Mace, 2008).

Navigating Airports and Transportation

Airports and other transportation hubs can be overwhelming, especially for senior travelers. However, with a few strategic tips, navigating these spaces can be much more manageable.

Using Airport Assistance Services: Most airports offer special assistance services for seniors, including wheelchair assistance, priority boarding, and help with luggage (U.S. Department of Transportation, 2021). These services can be requested when booking flights or by contacting the airline beforehand.

Packing Light and Using Rolling Luggage: Packing light can significantly reduce the physical strain of travel. Using a lightweight, rolling suitcase makes maneuvering through airports and hotels easier (Russell, 2013). Packing only the essentials and organizing your belongings in packing cubes or small bags can also help manage your luggage efficiently.

Booking Non-Stop Flights: Book non-stop flights whenever possible to reduce layover stress and the risk of missed connections (Goswami, 2008). Non-stop flights minimize travel time and the physical toll of getting on and off planes multiple times.

Arranging for Ground Transportation in Advance: To avoid the hassle of finding transportation after a long flight, arrange for ground transportation ahead of time. Many hotels offer shuttle services, or you can book a car service to pick you up at the airport (Rivers, 2005). This step can help you reach your destination comfortably and safely.

Enjoying the Journey

Traveling is not just about the destination but also about enjoying the journey. Ensuring comfort and entertainment can make travel more enjoyable and less stressful.

Bringing Along Comfort Items: Long trips can be tiring, so comfort items like a neck pillow, blanket, or compression socks can make the journey more pleasant (Zemp & Taylor, 2014). These items can help you rest better during flights or long drives.

Keeping Entertained with Books and Music: Pack a few books, magazines, or an e-reader loaded with your favorite titles. Music, audiobooks, and podcasts are great ways to pass the time and keep your mind engaged during the trip (Cassidy, 2007).

Staying Connected with Family via Smartphone Apps: Use smartphone apps to keep in touch with family and friends. Video calls, messaging apps, and travel journaling apps can help you share your experiences in real-time and keep you connected to loved ones, no matter where you are (Rainie & Wellman, 2012).

By planning your travel, maintaining health and safety, navigating transportation, and enjoying the journey, you can ensure a safe and enriching travel experience as a senior.

Journaling for Wellness: Tracking Your Health Journey

Benefits of Journaling

Journaling is a powerful tool for enhancing both mental and physical well-being. By regularly recording your thoughts, experiences, and health metrics, you can gain valuable insights into your behaviors and emotions, track your progress, and stay motivated on your wellness journey.

Enhancing Self-Awareness: One of the most significant benefits of journaling is enhancing self-awareness. When you write about your daily experiences, emotions, and health choices, you better understand your patterns, triggers, and behaviors. This self-awareness can lead to more informed decisions about your health and well-being (Pennebaker & Chung, 2011).

Tracking Progress and Setbacks: Journaling allows you to monitor your progress over time, whether working on improving your physical health, managing stress, or building new habits. Regularly documenting your efforts lets you see patterns and trends that might not be immediately apparent and can help you identify what works for you and where you need to make adjustments (Smyth, Stone, Hurewitz, & Kaell, 1999).

Reducing Stress and Anxiety: Writing about your thoughts and feelings can effectively manage stress and anxiety. Putting pen to paper (or fingers to keyboard) can help you process complex emotions, reduce mental clutter, and provide relief. Studies have shown that expressive writing can lower stress levels and improve emotional well-being (Baikie & Wilhelm, 2005).

Motivating Healthy Habits: Keeping a wellness journal can be a motivational tool, helping you stay on track with your health goals. By recording your successes, challenges, and goals, you create a tangible journey record that can inspire you to continue making positive changes (Cieslak, Benight, & Lehman, 2008).

Types of Wellness Journals

You can keep various types of wellness journals depending on your specific health goals and interests. Each journal serves a unique purpose and can help you focus on different aspects of your wellness journey.

Daily Health Logs: A daily health log is a straightforward way to track your overall health. You can record your physical activity, sleep patterns, hydration levels, and any symptoms or health changes you notice. This type of journal can help you identify patterns and correlations between your lifestyle choices and your health (Ochsner, 2010).

Gratitude Journals: A gratitude journal focuses on the positive aspects of your life, encouraging you to reflect on what you are thankful for each day. This practice enhances emotional well-being, increases life satisfaction, and promotes a positive outlook (Emmons & McCullough, 2003).

Exercise Journals: An exercise journal allows you to track your physical activity, including the type of exercise, duration, intensity, and how you felt afterward. This journal can help you monitor your fitness progress, set new goals, and stay motivated to maintain a regular exercise routine (Schutz, Gomer, & Munroe-Chandler, 2010).

Food Diaries: A food diary is valuable for those looking to improve their diet or manage specific health conditions. By recording what you eat and drink daily, you can become more mindful of your eating habits, identify triggers for unhealthy choices, and ensure that you meet your nutritional needs (Thompson & Subar, 2017).

Journaling Prompts

If you're new to journaling or need some inspiration to keep going, using prompts can be a helpful way to get started and maintain consistency. Here are a few prompts to consider for your wellness journal:

- **"What am I grateful for today?"** Reflecting on gratitude can help shift your focus from stress or challenges to the positive aspects of your life.

- **"How did I feel after my workout?"** Recording your post-exercise feelings can help you notice the immediate benefits of physical activity, reinforcing your motivation to stay active.

- **"What healthy meals did I enjoy this week?"** Tracking your meals can inspire you to continue making nutritious choices and discover new recipes you love.

Tips for Consistent Journaling

Maintaining a consistent journaling practice can be challenging, but with a few strategies, you can make it a rewarding and sustainable habit.

Setting a Regular Journaling Time: Choose a specific time to write in your journal daily. Whether in the morning as part of your daily routine or in the evening as a way to wind down, consistency is essential to making journaling a habit (Progoff, 1992).

Using a Dedicated Journal or App: A dedicated space for your entries, whether a physical journal or a digital app, can help you stay organized and focused. Many apps offer prompts, reminders, and customizable templates to suit your needs (Wright, 2011).

Reflecting on Entries Weekly or Monthly: Set aside time each week or month to review your journal entries. This reflection can help you identify patterns, celebrate progress, and adjust your goals as needed (Bolger, Davis, & Rafaeli, 2003).

Celebrating Progress and Milestones: Acknowledge and celebrate your achievements, no matter how small. Whether you've stuck to a new habit for a week or reached a significant health milestone, recognizing your progress can boost your motivation and confidence (Foster, 2012).

Journaling for wellness is a powerful tool for supporting mental and physical health. It can help you stay on track with your goals and maintain a positive outlook on your health journey.

CONCLUSION

As we reach the end of *Aging Like a Superstar*, it's clear that aging is not something to be feared but rather an opportunity to embrace life with renewed vigor and enthusiasm. The journey of aging gracefully is about more than maintaining physical appearance—it's about nurturing your mind, body, and spirit to live your best life at every stage.

By integrating the tips and strategies in this book, you've equipped yourself with the tools to shine in your golden years. Remember, the true essence of a superstar is not defined by youth but by the wisdom, experience, and authenticity that come with age.

Celebrate the skin you're in, cherish the memories you've made, and look forward to the possibilities that lie ahead. Aging like a superstar means owning your story, flaunting your uniqueness, and continuing to grow, learn, and love with each passing year. Your uniqueness is your strength, and it's something to be celebrated and cherished. The joy of reminiscing about your past, the laughter, the tears, the victories, and the lessons learned is a beautiful part of aging.

So, go forth confidently, embrace every wrinkle as a badge of honor, and let your inner superstar light up the world. Your future is filled with endless possibilities, and each day brings you closer to the best years of your life. The horizon is bright with hope and promise.

A REQUEST

If you have found value in this book, please share your experience by leaving a rating or a review on Amazon.

If you are reading an ebook, please click this link to be taken to your review page.

If you are reading a print book, point your phone's camera at the QR code below to be taken to your review page.

Thank you!

BIBLIOGRAPHY

ACSM (American College of Sports Medicine). (2009). American College of Sports Medicine position stand. Progression models in resistance training for healthy adults. *Medicine & Science in Sports & Exercise, 41*(3), 687-708.

Aitken, Z., Shrivastava, A., & Woolley, T. (2007). The effects of hair treatment and environmental conditions on hair quality. *International Journal of Cosmetic Science, 29*(5), 319-326.

Algoe, S. B., Gable, S. L., & Maisel, N. C. (2010). It's the little things: Everyday gratitude as a booster shot for romantic relationships. *Personal Relationships, 17*(2), 217-233.

Algoe, S. B., Haidt, J., & Gable, S. L. (2008). Beyond reciprocity: Gratitude and relationships in everyday life. *Emotion, 8*(3), 425-429.

Amberg, N., & Fogarassy, C. (2019). Green consumer behavior in the cosmetics market. *Sustainability, 11*(13), 3734.

Ammerman, N. T. (2014). *Sacred stories, spiritual tribes: Finding religion in everyday life.* Oxford University Press.

Anderson, R. B., & Burke, S. M. (2010). Stretching before exercise: An evidence-based approach. *Journal of Sports Medicine, 1*(1), 23-30.

Angelou, M. (1994). *Wouldn't take nothing for my journey now.* Random House.

Ashurst, J. V. (2017). Lemon water: A simple and effective remedy. *Nutrition Journal, 16*(1), 65-72.

Atchley, R. C. (1989). A continuity theory of normal aging. *The Gerontologist, 29*(2), 183-190.

Baikie, K. A., & Wilhelm, K. (2005). Emotional and physical health benefits of expressive writing. *Advances in Psychiatric Treatment, 11*(5), 338-346.

Bailey, R. (2005). Evaluating the relationship between physical education, sport, and social inclusion. *Educational Review, 57*(1), 71-90.

Bailey, R. (2015). The benefits of home-based exercise programs. *Journal of Physical Activity and Health, 12*(7), 938-943.

Baker, J. (2010). Participation in sport and exercise: Motivational factors for middle-aged and older adults. *Journal of Aging and Physical Activity, 18*(2), 177-196.

Baker, S. (2012). *Creative arts in counseling and mental health.* Sage.

Baker, S. (2012). *Celebrate your success: Positive reinforcement for health goals.* New York: Health Press.

Basset, R., & Leary, M. R. (1995). The need to belong: Desire for interpersonal attachments as a fundamental human motivation. *Psychological Bulletin, 117*(3), 497-529.

Bengtson, V. L. (2001). Beyond the nuclear family: The increasing importance of multigenerational bonds. *Journal of Marriage and Family, 63*(1), 1-16.

Bengen, W. P. (1994). Determining withdrawal rates using historical data. *Journal of Financial Planning, 7*(4), 171-180.

Berkman, L. F., Sheridan, S. L., Donahue, K. E., Halpern, D. J., & Crotty, K. (2011). Low health literacy and health outcomes: An updated systematic review. *Annals of Internal Medicine, 155*(2), 97-107.

Blanchett, D. M. (2013). Estimating the true cost of retirement. *Journal of Financial Planning, 26*(5), 51-60.

Booth, E., Bartlett, H. P., & Balfour, J. L. (2004). The role of teaching and mentoring in the development of a professional identity. *Studies in Higher Education, 29*(2), 241-261.

Booth, F. W., Roberts, C. K., & Laye, M. J. (2012). Lack of exercise is a major cause of chronic diseases. *Comprehensive Physiology, 2*(2), 1143-1211.

Bostock, S., Crosswell, A. D., Prather, A. A., & Steptoe, A. (2019). Mindfulness on-the-go: Effects of a mindfulness meditation app on work stress and well-being. *Journal of Occupational Health Psychology, 24*(1), 127-138.

Bouchard, G. (2014). How do parents react when their children leave home? An integrative review. *Journal of Adult Development, 21*(2), 69-79.

Bourgeault, C. (2004). *Centering prayer and inner awakening.* Cowley Publications.

Bravata, D. M., Smith-Spangler, C., Sundaram, V., Gienger, A. L., Lin, N., Lewis, R., ... & Sirard, J. R. (2007). Using pedometers to increase physical activity and improve health: A systematic review. *JAMA, 298*(19), 2296-2304.

Braithwaite, D. O., & Baxter, L. A. (2006). *Engaging theories in family communication: Multiple perspectives.* Sage.

Brown, K. W., & Ryan, R. M. (2003). The benefits of being present: Mindfulness and its role in psychological well-being. *Journal of Personality and Social Psychology, 84*(4), 822-848.

Bugos, J. A., Perlstein, W. M., McCrae, C. S., Brophy, T. S., & Bedenbaugh, P. H. (2007). Individualized piano instruction enhances executive functioning and working memory in older adults. *Aging & Mental Health, 11*(4), 464-471.

Campbell, H. A., & Törsleff, A. B. (2017). *Digital religion: Understanding religious practice in digital media.* Routledge.

Campbell, J. Y., & Viceira, L. M. (2002). *Strategic asset allocation: Portfolio choice for long-term investors.* Oxford University Press.

Carabotti, M., Scirocco, A., Maselli, M. A., & Severi, C. (2015). The gut-brain axis: Interactions between enteric microbiota, central and enteric nervous systems. *Annals of Gastroenterology, 28*(2), 203-209.

Carr, A. (2004). Positive psychology: The science of happiness and human strengths. *British Journal of Psychiatry, 184*(5), 475-476.

Carstensen, L. L. (1992). Social and emotional patterns in adulthood: Support for socioemotional selectivity theory. *Psychology and Aging, 7*(3), 331-338.

Carstensen, L. L., Isaacowitz, D. M., & Charles, S. T. (1999). Taking time seriously: A theory of socioemotional selectivity. *American Psychologist, 54*(3), 165-181.

Cassidy, J. (2007). The benefits of audiobooks for the elderly. *Journal of Aging Studies, 21*(4), 306-315.

Cavanagh, H. M., & Wilkinson, J. M. (2002). Biological activities of lavender essential oil. *Phytotherapy Research, 16*(4), 301-308.

Cherrier, H., & Pon, D. (2012). Recycling, reusing, and reducing: The role of the consumer in minimizing waste. *Journal of Consumer Behaviour, 11*(1), 38-47.

Chien, L. Y., Chu, H., Guo, J. L., Liao, Y. M., Chang, L. I., Chen, C. H., & Chou, K. R. (2011). Caregiver support groups in patients with dementia: A meta-analysis. *International Journal of Geriatric Psychiatry, 26*(10), 1089-1098.

Cieslak, R., Benight, C. C., & Lehman, V. C. (2008). Coping self-efficacy mediates the effects of negative cognitions on posttraumatic distress. *Behaviour Research and Therapy, 46*(7), 788-798.

Clarke, L. H., & Korotchenko, A. (2011). Aging and the body: A review. *Journal of Aging Studies, 25*(1), 1-10.

Cogley, R. M., Archambault, T. A., Fibeger, J. F., Koverman, J. W., Youdas, J. W., & Hollman, J. H. (2005). Comparison of muscle activation using various hand positions during the push-up exercise. *Journal of Strength and Conditioning Research, 19*(3), 628-633.

Cohen, G. D. (2006). Research on creativity and aging: The positive impact of the arts on health and illness. *Generations, 30*(1), 7-15.

Cohen, S., & Wills, T. A. (1985). Stress, social support, and the buffering hypothesis. *Psychological Bulletin, 98*(2), 310-357.

Cohen, S., Janicki-Deverts, D., & Miller, G. E. (2007). Psychological stress and disease. *JAMA, 298*(14), 1685-1687.

Collado, J. C., Tella, V., & Triplett, N. T. (2009). A method for monitoring intensity during aquatic resistance exercises. *Journal of Strength and Conditioning Research, 23*(6), 1756-1762.

Conrad, A., & Roth, W. T. (2007). Muscle relaxation therapy for anxiety disorders: It works but how? *Journal of Anxiety Disorders, 21*(3), 243-264.

Conrad, P., & Adams, C. (2012). The effects of clinical aromatherapy for anxiety and depression in the high-risk postpartum woman: A pilot study. *Complementary Therapies in Clinical Practice, 18*(3), 164-168.

Coyle, E. F. (2004). Fluid and fuel intake during exercise. *Journal of Sports Sciences, 22*(1), 39-55.

Craft, L. L., & Perna, F. M. (2004). The benefits of exercise for the clinically depressed. *Primary Care Companion to The Journal of Clinical Psychiatry, 6*(3), 104-111.

Csikszentmihalyi, M. (1996). *Creativity: Flow and the psychology of discovery and invention.* HarperCollins.

Csikszentmihalyi, M. (1997). *Finding flow: The psychology of engagement with everyday life.* Basic Books.

DeGarmo, M. T. (2010). *Starting your own book club: Ideas for creating great discussion groups.* Harlequin.

Doherty, K., & Feeney, J. A. (2004). The composition of attachment networks throughout the adult years. *Personal Relationships, 11*(4), 469-488.

Dunlop, T. (2017). The effective use of budgeting tools and apps for retirement planning. *Retirement Today Publishing.*

Dweck, C. S. (2006). *Mindset: The new psychology of success.* Random House.

Ellison, C. G., & Fan, D. (2008). Daily spiritual experiences and psychological well-being among US adults. *Social Indicators Research, 88*(2), 247-271.

Ellison, C. G., & George, L. K. (1994). Religious involvement, social ties, and social support in a southeastern community. *Journal for the Scientific Study of Religion, 33*(1), 46-61.

Emmons, R. A., & McCullough, M. E. (2003). Counting blessings versus burdens: An experimental investigation of gratitude and subjective well-being in daily life. *Journal of Personality and Social Psychology, 84*(2), 377-389.

Evangelista, M. T. P., Abad-Casintahan, F., & Lopez-Villafuerte, L. (2014). The effect of topical virgin coconut oil on SCORAD index, transepidermal water loss, and skin capacitance in mild to moderate pediatric atopic dermatitis: A randomized, double-blind, clinical trial. *International Journal of Dermatology, 53*(1), 100-108.

Ekor, M. (2014). The growing use of herbal medicines: Issues relating to adverse reactions and challenges in monitoring safety. *Frontiers in Pharmacology, 4*(177), 1-10.

Farnworth, E. R. (2005). Kefir—a complex probiotic. *Food Science and Technology Bulletin: Functional Foods, 2*(1), 1-17.

Foster, R. J. (1998). *Celebration of discipline: The path to spiritual growth.* Harper & Row.

Fredrickson, B. L. (2001). The role of positive emotions in positive psychology: The broaden-and-build theory of positive emotions. *American Psychologist, 56*(3), 218-226.

Fried, L. P. (2010). Strategies for promoting physical activity among older adults. *Journal of Aging and Health, 22*(5), 646-660.

Furman, R. (1997). *Wrinkles: Signs of aging or symbols of wisdom?* Perennial.

Giugliano, D., Ceriello, A., & Esposito, K. (2006). The effects of diet on inflammation: Emphasis on the metabolic syndrome. *Journal of the American College of Cardiology, 48*(4), 677-685.

Glover, M. (2011). *Finding peace in retirement: Spiritual practices for the golden years.* Crossway.

Goel, N., Kim, H., & Lao, R. P. (2005). An olfactory stimulus modifies nighttime sleep in young men and women. *Chronobiology International, 22*(5), 889-904.

Goyal, M., Singh, S., Sibinga, E. M., Gould, N. F., Rowland-Seymour, A., Sharma, R., ... & Haythornthwaite, J. A. (2014). Meditation programs for psychological stress and well-being: A systematic review and meta-analysis. *JAMA Internal Medicine, 174*(3), 357-368.

Greeson, J. M., Sanford, B., & Monti, D. A. (2001). St. John's wort (Hypericum perforatum): A review of the current pharmacological, toxicological, and clinical literature. *Psychopharmacology, 153*(4), 402-414.

Griffin, S. A., Jones, R., & Van Mechelen, W. (2014). Efficacy of an exercise program as intervention to reduce physical activity disparities. *Preventive Medicine, 67*(1), 129-135.

Gupta, S. C., Patchva, S., & Aggarwal, B. B. (2013). Therapeutic roles of curcumin: Lessons learned from clinical trials. *AAPS Journal, 15*(1), 195-218.

Guthrie, B. M., Brandt, E. J., & Lu, M. Y. (2015). Evaluating the potential health risks of exposure to endocrine-disrupting chemicals in personal care products. *Environmental Health Perspectives, 123*(9), A241-A245.

Hamer, M., & Chida, Y. (2008). Physical activity and risk of neurodegenerative disease: A systematic review of prospective evidence. *Psychological Medicine, 39*(1), 3-11.

Hartocollis, P. (2005). *Staying sane when you're parenting adult children.* Rodale.

Haskell, W. L., Lee, I. M., Pate, R. R., Powell, K. E., Blair, S. N., Franklin, B. A., ... & Bauman, A. (2007). Physical activity and public health: Updated recommendation for adults from the American College of Sports Medicine and the American Heart Association. *Medicine & Science in Sports & Exercise, 39*(8), 1423-1434.

Hepburn, A. (1991). *The beauty of a woman: Timeless elegance.* Chronicle Books.

Hertzog, C., Kramer, A. F., Wilson, R. S., & Lindenberger, U. (2008). Enrichment effects on adult cognitive development: Can the functional capacity of older adults be preserved and enhanced? *Psychological Science in the Public Interest, 9*(1), 1-65.

Hill, P. L., & Turiano, N. A. (2014). Purpose in life as a predictor of mortality across adulthood. *Psychological Science, 25*(7), 1482-1486.

Hofmann, S. G., Asnaani, A., Vonk, I. J., Sawyer, A. T., & Fang, A. (2012). The efficacy of cognitive behavioral therapy: A review of meta-analyses. *Cognitive Therapy and Research, 36*(5), 427-440.

Hongratanaworakit, T. (2011). Aroma-therapeutic effects of massage blended essential oils on humans. *Natural Product Communications, 6*(8), 1199-1204.

Holt-Lunstad, J., Smith, T. B., & Layton, J. B. (2010). Social relationships and mortality risk: A meta-analytic review. *PLOS Medicine, 7*(7), e1000316.

Jacobson, B. H., Boolani, A., & Smith, D. B. (2008). Changes in back pain, sleep quality, and perceived stress after introduction of new bedding systems. *Journal of Chiropractic Medicine, 7*(3), 94-100.

Jang, S. N., & Tang, F. (2016). Effects of social networks on the health of Korean older adults: Differences in age, gender, and life satisfaction. *Journal of Aging and Health, 28*(3), 363-384.

Jerath, R., Edry, J. W., Barnes, V. A., & Jerath, V. (2006). Physiology of long pranayamic breathing: Neural respiratory elements may provide a mechanism that explains how slow deep breathing shifts the autonomic nervous system. *Medical Hypotheses, 67*(3), 566-571.

Johnson, C. R., Mukhtar, H., & Ahmad, N. (2010). Green tea polyphenols as cancer chemopreventive agents. *Nutritional Cancer, 62*(7), 931-937.

Johnson, J. R., & Gannon, M. (2014). *Downsizing: How to simplify your life by reducing clutter and living without excess.* V. Publishing.

Keating, T. (2009). *Open mind, open heart: The contemplative dimension of the gospel.* Bloomsbury Publishing.

Keogh, J. W., Kilding, A., Pidgeon, P., Ashley, L., & Gillis, D. (2009). Physical benefits of dancing for healthy older adults: A review. *Journal of Aging and Physical Activity, 17*(4), 479-500.

Kinnafick, F. E., Thøgersen-Ntoumani, C., & Duda, J. L. (2014). Physical activity adoption to adherence, lapse, and dropout: A self-determination theory perspective. *Qualitative Health Research, 24*(5), 706-718.

Koenig, H. G. (2002). *The healing power of faith: Science explores medicine's last great frontier.* Simon & Schuster.

Koenig, H. G. (2012). *Spirituality in patient care: Why, how, when, and what.* Templeton Press.

Kolasinski, S. L., Neogi, T., Hochberg, M. C., Oatis, C., Guyatt, G., Block, J., & Toupin-April, K. (2020). 2019 American College of Rheumatology/Arthritis Foundation guideline for the management of osteoarthritis of the hand, hip, and knee. *Arthritis Care & Research, 72*(2), 149-162.

Kondo, M. (2014). *The life-changing magic of tidying up: The Japanese art of decluttering and organizing.* Ten Speed Press.

Koo, J. H. (2013). Coffee and health: A review of recent human research. *Critical Reviews in Food Science and Nutrition, 53*(6), 544-562.

Krishnan, S., Tokar, T. N., Boylan, M. M., Griffin, K., Feng, D., & McMurray, R. G. (2015). Zumba® dance improves health in overweight/obese or type 2 diabetic women. *American Journal of Health Behavior, 39*(1), 109-120.

Kraemer, W. J., Adams, K., Cafarelli, E., Dudley, G. A., Dooly, C., Feigenbaum, M. S., ... & McBride, J. M. (2002). American College of Sports Medicine position stand. Progression models in resistance training for healthy adults. *Medicine & Science in Sports & Exercise, 34*(2), 364-380.

Layne, J. E., & Nelson, M. E. (1999). The effects of progressive resistance training on bone density: A review. *Medicine & Science in Sports & Exercise, 31*(1), 25-30.

Lee, M. S., & Lee, J. A. (2014). Aromatherapy for health care: An overview of systematic reviews. *Maturitas, 79*(3), 179-185.

Lee, S., Kim, M., & Jung, E. (2013). Effects of green tea polyphenol (-)-epigallocatechin-3-gallate on skin mRNA expression of antioxidative enzymes. *Annals of Dermatology, 25*(2), 282-287.

Levin, J. (2001). *God, faith, and health: Exploring the spirituality-healing connection.* John Wiley & Sons.

Liu-Ambrose, T., Donaldson, M. G., Ahamed, Y., Graf, P., Cook, W. L., Close, J., & Lord, S. R. (2004). Otago home-based strength and balance retraining improves executive functioning and gait in older adults: A cluster randomized controlled trial. *Journal of the American Geriatrics Society, 56*(10), 1821-1830.

Locke, E. A., & Latham, G. P. (2002). Building a practically useful theory of goal setting and task motivation: A 35-year odyssey. *American Psychologist, 57*(9), 705-717.

Luthar, S. S., Cicchetti, D., & Becker, B. (2000). The construct of resilience: A critical evaluation and guidelines for future work. *Child Development, 71*(3), 543-562.

Mach, N., & Fuster-Botella, D. (2017). Endurance exercise and gut microbiota: A review. *Journal of Sport and Health Science, 6*(2), 179-197.

Majewski, D. A. (2014). Honey in dermatology and skin care: A review. *Journal of Cosmetic Dermatology, 13*(2), 178-184.

Manini, T. M. (2010). Energy expenditure and physical activity in older adults. *American Journal of Clinical Nutrition, 91*(3), 739-746.

Marco, M. L., Sanders, M. E., Gänzle, M., Arrieta, M. C., Cotter, P. D., De Vuyst, L., ... & Hill, C. (2017). The International Scientific Association for Probiotics and Prebiotics (ISAPP) consensus statement on fermented foods. *Nature Reviews Gastroenterology & Hepatology, 14*(4), 196-208.

Maslach, C., & Leiter, M. P. (2016). Understanding the burnout experience: Recent research and its implications for psychiatry. *World Psychiatry, 15*(2), 103-111.

McCabe, S., & Johnson, S. (2013). The happiness factor in tourism: Subjective well-being and social tourism. *Annals of Tourism Research, 41*(1), 42-65.

McCarthy, M. F. (2012). Nutritional modulation of skin aging and skin sensitivity: Focus on inflammation, glycation, and mitochondrial dysfunction. *Journal of Clinical and Aesthetic Dermatology, 5*(9), 29-36.

McEwen, B. S. (2006). Protective and damaging effects of stress mediators: Central role of the brain. *Dialogues in Clinical Neuroscience, 8*(4), 367-381.

McEwen, B. S. (2007). Physiology and neurobiology of stress and adaptation: Central role of the brain. *Physiological Reviews, 87*(3), 873-904.

McFarland, L. V. (2015). From yaks to yogurt: The history, development, and current use of probiotics. *Clinical Infectious Diseases, 60*(S2), S85-S90.

McMahon, S. B. (2011). The role of dry skin brushing in health promotion: A literature review. *Complementary Therapies in Clinical Practice, 17*(4), 220-225.

Miller, C. K., Kristeller, J. L., Headings, A., & Nagaraja, H. (2012). Comparison of a mindful eating intervention to a diabetes self-management intervention among adults with type 2 diabetes: A randomized controlled trial. *Health Education & Behavior, 39*(4), 536-545.

Miller, M. J. S., & Shukitt-Hale, B. (2012). Berry fruit enhances beneficial signaling in the brain. *Journal of Agricultural and Food Chemistry, 60*(23), 5709-5715.

Mitchell, B. A., & Lovegreen, L. D. (2009). The empty nest syndrome in midlife families: A multimethod exploration of parental gender differences and cultural dynamics. *Journal of Family Issues, 30*(12), 1651-1670.

Monteiro, C. A., Cannon, G., Levy, R. B., Moubarac, J. C., Jaime, P., Martins, A. P., ... & Canella, D. (2018). Ultra-processed foods: What they are and how to identify them. *Public Health Nutrition, 21*(1), 1-6.

Moss, M., Hewitt, S., & Moss, L. (2012). Modulation of cognitive performance and mood by aromas of peppermint and ylang-ylang. *International Journal of Neuroscience, 118*(1), 59-77.

Mozaffarian, D., & Wu, J. H. Y. (2012). Omega-3 fatty acids and cardiovascular disease: Effects on risk factors, molecular pathways, and clinical events. *Journal of the American College of Cardiology, 58*(20), 2047-2067.

Neff, K. D. (2003). The development and validation of a scale to measure self-compassion. *Self and Identity, 2*(3), 223-250.

Nguyen, T. A., Friedman, A. J., & Papathakis, P. (2014). Avocado and other botanical and herbal products with effects on hair and scalp. *Journal of Cosmetic Dermatology, 13*(2), 146-153.

Northouse, L. L., Katapodi, M. C., Song, L., Zhang, L., & Mood, D. W. (2012). Interventions with family caregivers of cancer patients: Meta-analysis of randomized trials. *CA: A Cancer Journal for Clinicians, 60*(5), 317-339.

O'Hara, K. (2008). Understanding geocaching practices and motivations. *Conference on Human Factors in Computing Systems, 10*(1), 1177-1186.

Oja, P., Titze, S., Bauman, A., de Geus, B., Krenn, P., Reger-Nash, B., & Kohlberger, T. (2011). Health benefits of cycling: A systematic review. *Scandinavian Journal of Medicine & Science in Sports, 21*(4), 496-509.

O'Keefe, J. H., Gheewala, N. M., & O'Keefe, J. O. (2008). Dietary strategies for improving post-prandial glucose, lipids, inflammation, and cardiovascular health. *Journal of the American College of Cardiology, 51*(3), 249-255.

Page, P. (2012). Current concepts in muscle stretching for exercise and rehabilitation. *International Journal of Sports Physical Therapy, 7*(1), 109-119.

Park, D. C., & Bischof, G. N. (2013). The aging mind: Neuroplasticity in response to cognitive training. *Dialogues in Clinical Neuroscience, 15*(1), 109-119.

Pargament, K. I. (2007). *Spiritually integrated psychotherapy: Understanding and addressing the sacred.* Guilford Press.

Pate, R. R., Trost, S. G., Felton, G. M., Ward, D. S., Dowda, M., & Saunders, R. (1997). Correlates of physical activity behavior in rural youth. *Research Quarterly for Exercise and Sport, 68*(3), 241-248.

Pennebaker, J. W. (1997). *Opening up: The healing power of expressing emotions.* Guilford Press.

Pennebaker, J. W., & Chung, C. K. (2011). Expressive writing: Connections to physical and mental health. In H. S. Friedman (Ed.), *The Oxford handbook of health psychology* (pp. 417-437). Oxford University Press.

Pfau, W. D. (2013). A broader framework for determining an efficient retirement income strategy. *Journal of Financial Planning, 26*(2), 44-51.

Popkin, B. M., D'Anci, K. E., & Rosenberg, I. H. (2010). Water, hydration, and health. *Nutrition Reviews, 68*(8), 439-458.

Progoff, I. (1992). *At a journal workshop: Writing to access the power of the unconscious and evoke creative ability.* New York: Tarcher.

Putnam, R. D. (2000). *Bowling alone: The collapse and revival of American community.* Simon & Schuster.

Rao, R. K., & Samak, G. (2012). Role of glutamine in protection of intestinal epithelial tight junctions. *Journal of Epithelial Biology & Pharmacology, 5*(1), 47-54.

Reiche, E. M., Nunes, S. O., & Morimoto, H. K. (2004). Stress, depression, the immune system, and cancer. *The Lancet Oncology, 5*(10), 617-625.

Rele, A. S., & Mohile, R. B. (2003). Effect of mineral oil, sunflower oil, and coconut oil on prevention of hair damage. *Journal of Cosmetic Science, 54*(2), 175-192.

Ridker, P. M., & Luscher, T. F. (2014). Anti-inflammatory therapies for cardiovascular disease. *European Heart Journal, 35*(27), 1782-1791.

Roberfroid, M. (2007). Prebiotics: The concept revisited. *The Journal of Nutrition, 137*(3), 830S-837S.

Rogers, C., & Jarrett, C. (2007). The importance of travel insurance for senior citizens. *Travel Medicine and Infectious Disease, 5*(1), 60-65.

Ross, R., Dagnone, D., Jones, P. J., Smith, H., Paddags, A., Hudson, R., & Janssen, I.

(2000). Reduction in obesity and related comorbid conditions after diet-induced weight loss or exercise-induced weight loss in men: A randomized, controlled trial. *Annals of Internal Medicine, 133*(2), 92-103.

Scheer, F. A., Hilton, M. F., Mantzoros, C. S., & Shea, S. A. (2010). Adverse metabolic and cardiovascular consequences of circadian misalignment. *Proceedings of the National Academy of Sciences, 106*(11), 4453-4458.

Schellenberg, E. G. (2004). Music lessons enhance IQ. *Psychological Science, 15*(8), 511-514.

Schlicht, J., Camaione, D. N., & Owen, S. V. (2001). Effect of intense strength training on standing balance, walking speed, and sit-to-stand performance in older adults. *The Journals of Gerontology Series A: Biological Sciences and Medical Sciences, 56*(5), M281-M286.

Schoenfeld, B. J. (2010). The mechanisms of muscle hypertrophy and their application to resistance training. *Journal of Strength and Conditioning Research, 24*(10), 2857-2872.

Shearer, C., & Moss, M. (2015). *The complete guide to downsizing and decluttering: Real life advice and solutions for moving on.* House & Home Publishing.

Sherman, K. J., Wellman, R. D., Cook, A. J., Cherkin, D. C., & Ceballos, R. M. (2011). Mediators of yoga and stretching for chronic low back pain. *Evidence-Based Complementary and Alternative Medicine, 2011*, 1-10.

Slavin, J. (2013). Fiber and prebiotics: Mechanisms and health benefits. *Nutrients, 5*(4), 1417-1435.

Srivastava, J. K., Shankar, E., & Gupta, S. (2010). Chamomile: A herbal medicine of the past with a bright future (review). *Molecular Medicine Reports, 3*(6), 895-901.

Steinemann, A. (2017). Health and societal effects from exposure to fragranced consumer products. *Preventive Medicine Reports, 5*(1), 45-47.

Stevens, J. A., Mahoney, J. E., Ehrenreich, H., & Parsons, S. (2012). Preventing falls in older adults: Recommendations for pharmacy personnel and pharmacists. *Journal of the American Pharmacists Association, 52*(3), 360-367.

Stern, Y. (2009). Cognitive reserve. *Neuropsychologia, 47*(10), 2015-2028.

Streeter, C. C., Gerbarg, P. L., Saper, R. B., Ciraulo, D. A., & Brown, R. P. (2012). Effects of yoga on the autonomic nervous system, gamma-aminobutyric-acid, and allostasis in epilepsy, depression, and post-traumatic stress disorder. *Medical Hypotheses, 78*(5), 571-579.

Stuckey, H. L., & Nobel, J. (2010). The connection between art, healing, and public health: A review of current literature. *American Journal of Public Health, 100*(2), 254-263.

Surjushe, A., Vasani, R., & Saple, D. G. (2008). Aloe vera: A short review. *Indian Journal of Dermatology, 53*(4), 163-166.

Thigpen, C. A., Padua, D. A., Michener, L. A., Guskiewicz, K. M., Giuliani, C., Keener, J. D., & Stergiou, N. (2010). Head and shoulder posture affect scapular mechanics and muscle activity in overhead tasks. *Journal of Electromyography and Kinesiology, 20*(4), 701-709.

Thompson, M. (2012). *Soul feast: An invitation to the Christian spiritual life.* Westminster

John Knox Press.

Thoma, M. V., La Marca, R., Brönnimann, R., Finkel, L., Ehlert, U., & Nater, U. M. (2013). The effect of music on the human stress response. *PLoS ONE, 8*(8), e70156.

Tisserand, R., & Young, R. (2013). *Essential oil safety: A guide for health care professionals.* Elsevier Health Sciences.

Tudor-Locke, C., Craig, C. L., Brown, W. J., Clemes, S. A., de Cocker, K., Giles-Corti, B., ... & Blair, S. N. (2011). How many steps/day are enough? For adults. *International Journal of Behavioral Nutrition and Physical Activity, 8*(1), 1-17.

Tugade, M. M., & Fredrickson, B. L. (2004). Resilient individuals use positive emotions to bounce back from negative emotional experiences. *Journal of Personality and Social Psychology, 86*(2), 320-333.

Verghese, J., Lipton, R. B., Katz, M. J., Hall, C. B., Derby, C. A., Kuslansky, G., ... & Buschke, H. (2003). Leisure activities and the risk of dementia in the elderly. *New England Journal of Medicine, 348*(25), 2508-2516.

Vogt, N. M., Romano, K. A., Darst, B. F., Engelman, C. D., Johnson, S. C., Carlsson, C. M., ... & Bendlin, B. B. (2017). The gut microbiota-derived metabolite trimethylamine N-oxide is elevated in Alzheimer's disease. *Alzheimer's Research & Therapy, 9*(1), 1-8.

Vogt, N. M., Romano, K. A., Darst, B. F., Engelman, C. D., Johnson, S. C., Carlsson, C. M., ... & Bendlin, B. B. (2017). The gut microbiota-derived metabolite trimethylamine N-oxide is elevated in Alzheimer's disease. *Alzheimer's Research & Therapy, 9*(1), 1-8.

Wan, C. Y., & Schlaug, G. (2010). Music making as a tool for promoting brain plasticity across the life span. *The Neuroscientist, 16*(5), 566-577.

Warburton, D. E., Nicol, C. W., & Bredin, S. S. (2006). Health benefits of physical activity: The evidence. *CMAJ, 174*(6), 801-809.

Wheeler, J., & Watkins, E. (1988). A review of yoga as a therapeutic intervention. *Orthopaedic Nursing, 7*(1), 36-39.

Willard, D. (2002). *Renovation of the heart: Putting on the character of Christ.* NavPress.

Wood, A. M., Froh, J. J., & Geraghty, A. W. (2010). Gratitude and well-being: A review and theoretical integration. *Clinical Psychology Review, 30*(7), 890-905.

Woronuk, G., Demissie, Z., Rheault, M., & Mahmoud, S. (2011). Biosynthesis and therapeutic properties of frankincense essential oil. *Planta Medica, 77*(11), 1115-1126.

Wright, N. T. (2010). *Scripture and the authority of God: How to read the Bible today.* HarperOne.

Youkhana, S., Dean, C. M., Wolff, M., Sherrington, C., & Tiedemann, A. (2016). Yoga-based exercise improves balance and mobility in people aged 60 and over: A systematic review and meta-analysis. *Age and Ageing, 45*(1), 21-29.

Zeidan, F., Johnson, S. K., Diamond, B. J., David, Z., & Goolkasian, P. (2010). Mindfulness meditation improves cognition: Evidence of brief mental training. *Consciousness and Cognition, 19*(2), 597-605.

Zhou, X., Ferguson, S. A., Matthews, R. W., Sargent, C., Darwent, D., & Kennaway, D. J. (2017). Sleep, wake and phase dependent effects of caffeine on sleep and vigilance in shift workers. *Journal of Sleep Research, 26*(3), 380-385.

ABOUT THE AUTHOR

Elliott Middleton, PhD, is a former university professor and decision scientist with some of the world's largest financial institutions. He lives with his family in Tennessee.

www.ingramcontent.com/pod-product-compliance
Lightning Source LLC
Chambersburg PA
CBHW071943150726
47999CB00001B/299